The Transplant Handbook

Your Kidney Transplant Journey: Preparation to Post-Op

John Carter

Patient, Survivor

Published by The Wisdom Grove, LLC
Battle Creek, Michigan
www.thewisdomgrove.org

ISBN 978-0-9791947-1-9 - Paperback
ISBN 978-0-9791947-2-6 - ebook

First Edition

Portions of this book, including text and images, were created, edited or refined with the assistance of artificial intelligence tools. All content remains under the creative direction and authorship of the writer.

DEDICATION

To everyone whose life was interrupted by a disease they never asked for — and to those who love.

To my donor — whose life was cut short, yet whose gifts lives on. His family's generosity can never erase their grief, and those of us saved by his many donations could never say "thank you" enough to equal what we received.

It would be impossible to name every individual who helped along the way, but those most crucial on the journey include: **Sharon, Theresa, Rex, John, Savannah, Sara, Carrie, Heather.**

About the cover: The illustration is to convey the crossing of the bridge for the darkness of dialysis treatments to the light, freedoms and joy of live after a transplant.

Author's Note

There's no handbook for hearing the words *end-stage renal disease*. There's no calm, no clarity—just fear, confusion, and a thousand questions that no one seems ready to answer.

This book was born from the storm I went through. It's part practical guide, part personal story, and wholly meant to make your road just a little easier. I've been where you are—on dialysis, chasing appointments, weighing transplant options, trying to live while just trying to survive. This isn't a jelly-filled donut pep talk. It's real talk from someone who's been through the fire and found a way out the other side.

If you've just been diagnosed with ESRD, are waiting for a kidney, or are trying to wrap your head around the whole process —this book is for you. A transplant is not just survivable. It's doable. And you don't have to do it alone.

This is also the book your family and loved ones must read. They are on the journey with you. They will have their own reservations, their own concerns, their own questions.

You are only as smart as you are educated

- Unknown

Table of Contents

I: Before the Journey Begins

"You can't go back and change the beginning, but you can start where you are and change the ending."
— C.S. Lewis

This opening section sets the stage for what lies ahead. It offers a personal introduction, clarifies important disclaimers, and provides the essential background to help you understand the full scope of the transplant journey before it even begins.

Chapters in this section:

Chapter 1 - Before We Begin: A Personal Note

Let me be clear from the start. I'm not here to talk anyone into or out of getting a transplant. That is deeply personal — one that only *you* can make.

You'll want to consult with yourself, your close friends and family, trusted medical professionals, dialysis technicians you may have grown close to, social workers, clergy or spiritual counselors.

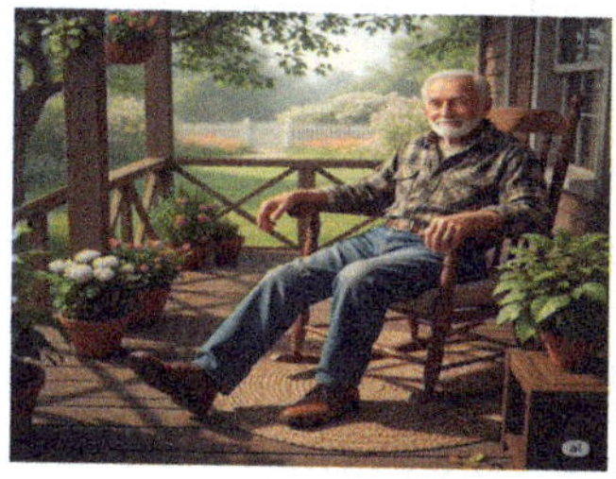

If you are on in-clinic dialysis, ask the staff or your kidney doctor if they can have any previous transplant patients contact you. I will share my story - but every story is different. The opinions of five or six or ???? more can provide you with additional insights and knowledge.

I want to give you fair warning: At times, I'm going to be blunt. Sometimes brutally so. That might make a few people uncomfortable. Sometimes the truth hurts. Most of the time it helps.

What you'll get here is raw honesty. Mixed with off the cuff, sometimes dry humor.

I won't sugarcoat what I lived through. I don't believe you'll benefit from hearing only rosy, ride-off-into-the-sunset stories. There are plenty of those stories. Sometimes, you have to weather some stormy weather and mountain passes before the easier times arrive.

I asked a lot of questions. But not enough. I considered many outcomes — yet overlooked others. I spoke to many people — but should've spoken to more. That's what this is all about: to help you dig a little deeper, be better prepared.

After reading this, I want you to challenge everything you have read. Not to prove me wrong - which you might - but so you have more knowledge, better understanding.

Ask questions. Question the answers. Ask questions about the answers you receive. Question the answers from "keyboard experts." If you don't fully understand, push until you do.

Please re-read the above paragraph at least 3 times. <u>Out loud!</u>

I was told I had a 1% chance of transplant failure. I was also told some patients heal slower than average. What they didn't say was how hard it could hit if you are *you're* an exception.

In my case, some of my healing complications were due to medical decisions, others simply fate. But the experience was real. It left a mark. At times I questioned why I signed up for a transplant. But now - I know why I did it. I am thrilled I did.

Throughout this book, I'll share parts of my personal journey to illustrate what a transplant patient might go through. Not because my story is special — but because real examples stick better than sterile "informational" text. I hope my story will give you a foundation to ask better questions and advocate for yourself more effectively. You are your own best friend.

By the time you read this, new procedures, policies, medications, and treatment options ~~may~~ will exist. But the emotional and decision-making aspects of this journey? Those don't change.

Whether you choose transplant, stay on dialysis, or pursue another path — I want nothing but the best for you. I truly do.

John Carter

Chapter 2 - Important Disclaimers

(or, Why You Should Still Listen to Your Doctor)

Before we dive in, here are a few points I need to say upfront:

1. **I am not a doctor.** I don't even play one on TV. I'm just a guy who's been through it and wants to help others by sharing what I learned. Your medical team—those folks with years of schooling, lab coats, and very serious expressions—are the real experts. This book is a companion, not a substitute. Use it to spark questions and curiosity, not replace professional advice.

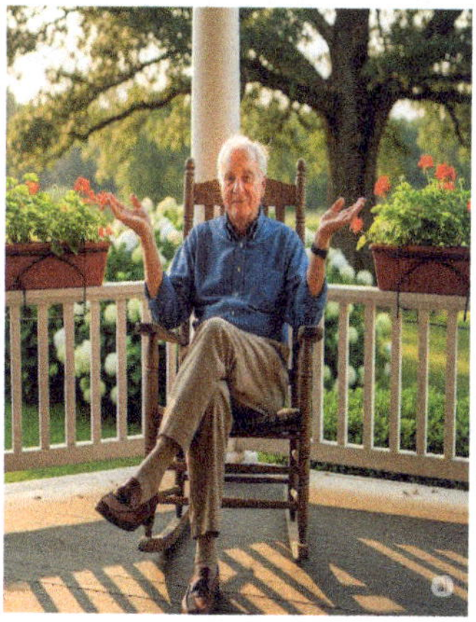

2. **Medicine changes fast.** What was true in 2020 (my transplant) might already be old news. New techniques, treatments, and studies are always rolling out. So if your doctor says something that doesn't match what's in here—please believe *them* and not the guy with the laptop. Or some social media post.

3. **Your prescriptions will be different than mine.** I will not list the exact medications I take. Your combo will be tailored to you. Just know what you're prescribed depends on your overall health, your doctor's recommendations, and what's new on the pharmacy shelf.

4. **Not everything is the same everywhere.** Believe it or not, transplant procedures can vary depending on where you live—even within the U.S. I'm still scratching my head over that one. So don't be surprised if something works a little differently in your state or region. (Again: see Disclaimer #1.)

5. **The future is coming—and it's bionic.** Artificial kidneys are in development and could change everything. Someday, parts of this book may feel like reading about rotary phones. Some things—like wound care and recovery—will still apply, the transplant world is shifting fast.

6. **Final word:** When in doubt, go back to Disclaimer #1. Seriously, highlight and underline it.

Chapter 3 - Background

In December 2008, my kidneys called it quits. Just packed up and walked off the job. The official diagnosis? End Stage Renal Disease—aka total kidney failure. Without jumping into hemodialysis three times a week, the outcome would've been, well... not ideal. So, I did what any stubborn, life-loving person would do—I started treatment. Because, well, not dying seemed like a solid Plan A.

Almost immediately, the doctors started tossing around the "T-word": transplant - like it was a casual weekend project.

For years, a mix of hurdles kept transplant off the table. Insurance requirements, aftercare plans (I had no one who could provide a month of care), and, oh yeah—I ran my own one-man business. A business that had consumed all my savings and actually put me in debt starting it up.

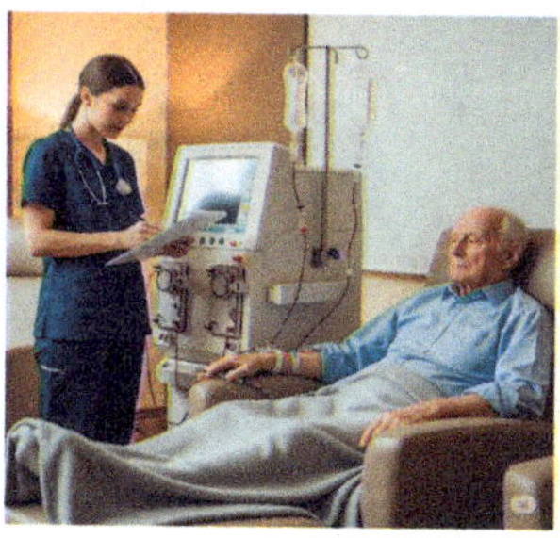

Fast forward to July 2013: plot twist. The shopping center where my little mail/shipping business lived got sold. The new landlord came in like a Monopoly villain and hiked my rent from $1,400 to $2,400 a month. That's not a typo.

It felt less like a rent increase, more like a ransom note. It was not sustainable for a one-man shop. Moving the store was out—too expensive, too risky. I knew I'd lose a big chunk of my regulars. Especially the mailbox crowd, which made up a hefty slice of the pie. The business could not afford a loss of as much as 40-50% of it's income and remain open. So I shut down, transferring customers to other businesses.

Now income-less and soon homeless, I did what made the most sense: I moved to Michigan to stay with family. New state, new dialysis clinic, new care team... and, yep, new transplant conversations. Mentally, I still wasn't there.

In early 2015, I returned to Las Vegas for a bit (sunshine has its perks) to try to re-establish myself financially. But in late 2017, I found myself back in Michigan for round two.

By now, dialysis was routine, and I'd become a human pin cushion. Right before moving, my graft blew out—great timing—so I was back to using a permacath in my chest.

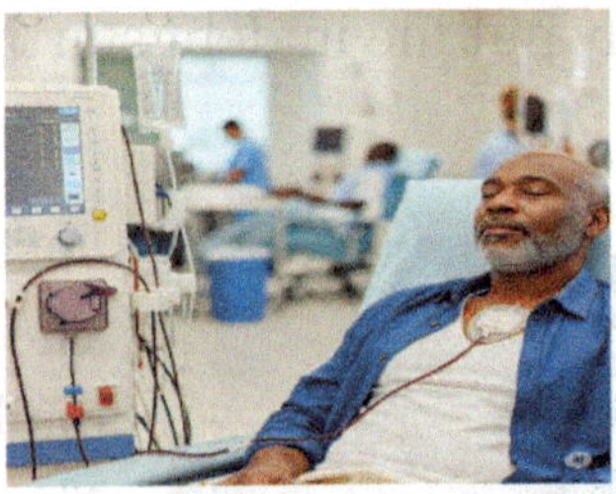

In February 2018, they installed a new graft in my left arm. It worked, kind of. The graft itself was fine, but the vein connection in the elbow decided to play games. Three outpatient procedures later (and one more looming by mid-2019), I started to question if this thing in my arm was a ticking time bomb.

That's when the mental scales started tipping. I was more afraid of another failed graft than of transplant surgery. And that is saying something. So, I told my clinic's social worker I was ready to explore options.

Following a meeting between the social worker, the dietitian, my sister (a.k.a. support team captain) and I - I agreed it was time to talk transplant.

My nephrologist agreed to send a referral to the University of Michigan Hospital transplant center.

At that point, I had 11 years of dialysis under my belt. If I got accepted, I'd be near the top of the list.

If I was accepted.

Chapter 4 - Understanding the Journey Ahead

Knowledge lights the path for you,
but it's education that teaches you how to walk it.

If you're reading this, you're probably overwhelmed, confused, or even scared. That's normal.

I've been where you are. I've walked the paths you're about to walk. My family and friends have traveled the roads your family and loved ones must also navigate. I'm someone who lived with kidney failure for more than 11 years. I survived hemodialysis. I endured the transplant process — including **two** post-op infections. And I came out the other side with a renewed life.

I compare the journey from dialysis to transplant to hiking Mount Everest. Thankfully, others have blazed the trail before you. You'll be assisted by guides, helpers, and support teams. Some will only be there at the start. Others will walk beside you the whole way. But all of them will cheer when you reach the summit.

Your story is unique. The circumstances that brought you here are different from from all others. But the questions you have? Others have asked them too. The fears you feel? Others have felt those as well. And the confusion clouding your thoughts? You're not alone in that fog.

From 2020 to 2024, nearly 130,000 kidney transplants were performed in the U.S. You are not walking this road in isolation. Yes, your path may feel daunting. But it is possible.

Think back to how drastically life changed when you began dialysis. The shift after transplant will be just as dramatic — maybe even more so. Once you've lost freedom, you understand just how precious it is. And once it's restored, it feels even sweeter.

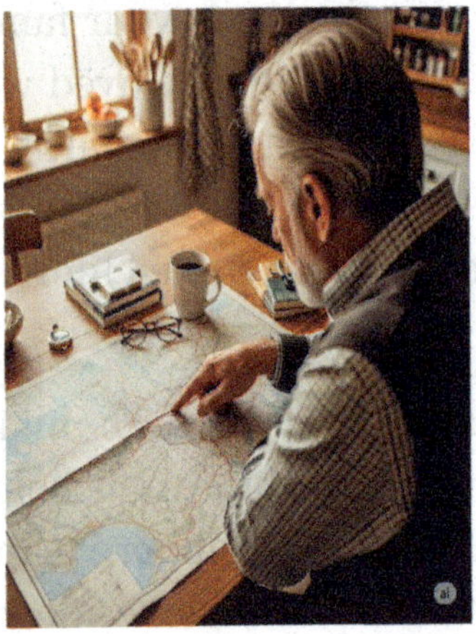

Why did I write this book? Because I needed it years ago. A clear, straightforward, easy-to-read guide. Yes, there was Facebook groups and forums. Yet information is scattered, biased, or unclear. This is the book I wish someone gave me: clear, straightforward, and grounded in experience.

In the pages ahead, I'll share what to expect, steps to take, how to prepare legally and financially, things to consider for housing and aftercare, and much more. I want to help you map your course to a new you.

The choice to pursue a transplant — to finish testing, go on the waiting list, and accept a kidney — is deeply personal. My aspiration is that this information helps you clear some of the fog, provides practical tools, and reassures you that a transplant isn't just possible — it's survivable.

Your transplant journey's gonna be a mixed bag, kind of like life out here in the sticks. Some days it'll feel like you're strapped into the Scrambler at the county fair, hangin' on for dear life.

Other days it's a long, flat stretch of Texas highway—nothing much happening but the hum of the tires and your own thoughts.

And then there'll be nights when it's more like a twisty two-lane road through the Tennessee mountains in the dark—you'll be squintin' and hopin' the next curve doesn't hold a surprise.

But here's the thing: on the other side of all that, there's a sunrise waitin' that'll knock your socks off, the kind that makes you stop, breathe deep, and say, "Well, that was worth the ride."

If you're feeling stuck, go talk to yourself. Seriously. You'd be amazed what future-you already knows.

II: Getting Transplant Ready

"The future belongs to those who prepare for it today."
— Malcolm X

This section prepares you for the many moving parts of transplant readiness—medical, legal, financial, and emotional. From the screening process to getting "the call," you'll gain insights that will help you plan wisely, protect yourself, and stay focused through a complicated but critical stage.

Chapters in this section:

Chapter 1 - The Screening Process: What to Expect

You don't need to know everything,
just enough to ask the right questions.

Transplant candidates go through a series of screenings. The types of screenings, the methods used, and the order they are completed are specific to the individual. The transplant team decides which tests are needed based on each patient's situation. And just to keep things fun, sometimes one screening's results lead to another test. And another.

Rather than just rattle off a list of possible tests, partially because I don't know everything they might come up with, I figured I'd walk you through *my* screening experience.

1.1 - My Screening Story

In August 2019, I traveled with my niece—my designated healthcare proxy - to the University of Michigan Hospital in Ann Arbor. It was a full-day affair, starting at 9 AM and wrapping up around 5 PM, not counting the two-hour drive each way. We did reward ourselves with a steak dinner at Texas Roadhouse afterward (unpaid plug), so at least the day ended on a high note.

1.1.1 - Arrived

After check in, I thought I would relax in the waiting room. I was wrong. A nurse came to get me and we walked about 50 feet to a testing station. First up: the basics: blood pressure, temperature, pulse, and weight.

Then came the infamous **walk test**. I was asked to walk about 15 feet briskly... to prove I could walk 15 feet briskly. Twice. Down and back.

This came *after* I'd already walked likely 1000 steps from the parking garage to the clinic and then about 50 feet from the waiting room to the vitals station, and another 75 feet down the hallway to where the 15' test took place.

Yeah, I thought the same thing you're probably thinking right now. I asked the nurse why those first 125 feet didn't count. She didn't have a good answer.

Guess she was paid by the step.

1.1.2 - Then Came the Needles...

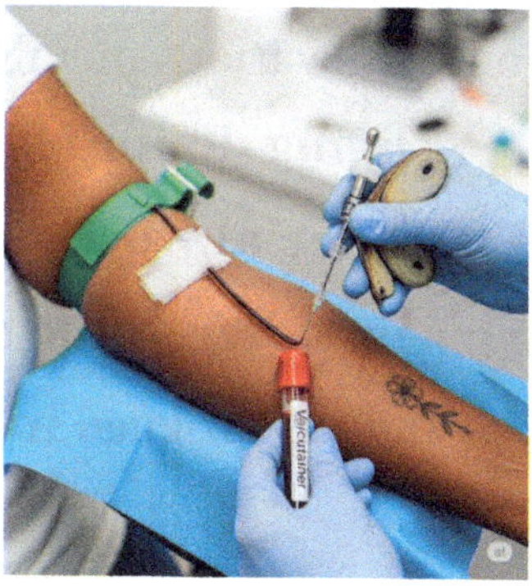

Next stop: **blood draw**. Around 10 vials, for blood typing, disease screening, general labs, and to create a baseline for future comparisons. The lady was required to draw from two different access points. Something about making sure there was no contamination by matching samples from the two sources. One right arm - one left arm.

Then a quick **upper body & chest X-ray**.

1.1.3 Group Meeting

The middle of the day involved a group session with other potential transplant candidates and their support people. Eight, maybe nine, transplant applicants were in the room. A nurse and a social worker from the transplant team joined us to explain the steps and procedures. We received a hefty info packet full of FAQs, forms, and general guidance. Hate to insult U of M Transplant, I had more questions after reading the book than I had before.

At least we got a sack lunch.

1.1.4 Private Meetings

The last part of the day was spent in an exam room meeting one-on-one with various members of the transplant team:

- a **living donor coordinator**
- the **social worker** (again, but this time privately)
- a **member of the surgical team**
- and my assigned **in-hospital nephrologist**

After that, we were done for the day being given the instructions *"don't call us we will call you"*.

2.1.4.1 - A Quick Story

While chatting with the living transplant coordinator, he asked if I had approached any family members about donating.

I replied, *"My Family? What makes you think I can get a body part? I have trouble getting a ride to the airport—even when I offer to pay for gas and buy lunch!"*

My niece laughing—enthusiastically agreed.

Your results with family may vary.

1.3 - More Tests? Of Course There Were...

The following week, the transplant team held a case review to go over every candidate's results. My review led to the following "bonus round" of testing:

- A heart stress test (FYI: past romantic heartbreaks did *not* count regardless of my heartaches)
- An ultrasound of my lower abdominal area
- An upper and lower GI series

1.3.1 - A Stress Test... That Was Stressful

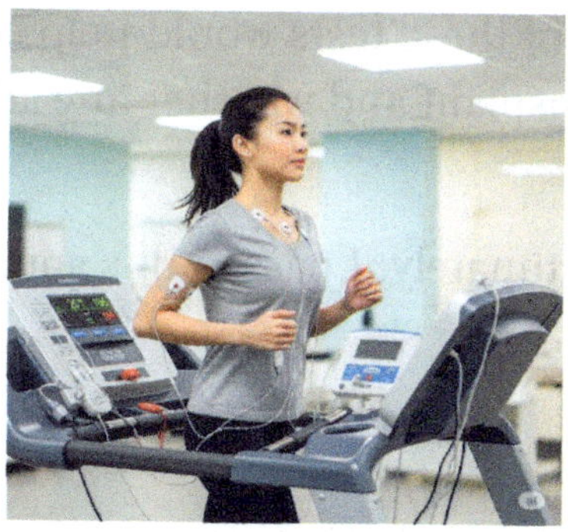

My heart stress test was chemical, not on a treadmill or other *physical exertion method.*

At one point, the pain got so intense I was practically begging them to stop.

Thankfully, they had enough "pictures" at that point and ended it

1.3.2 - The abdominal ultrasound

The ultrasound was used to check for a suitable spot to place the new kidney. For those curious—your old kidneys are usually left in place unless they pose a health risk. This was the only test that was close to my home – about 10 minutes vs an hour or more for each of the other two.

1.3.3 - Upper and lower GI series

If you know, you know. Nothing else to discuss. Thankfully, I got to sleep during the procedure. :)

All of these tests would help confirm if I was physically ready for transplant and whether any additional testing was needed.

Fortunately, I passed this gauntlet and didn't need any more.

1.4 - A Little Tooth Trouble

I already knew I had a partially impacted lower right wisdom tooth poking out of my jaw. This would be flagged as a possible infection source—something you don't want after a transplant.

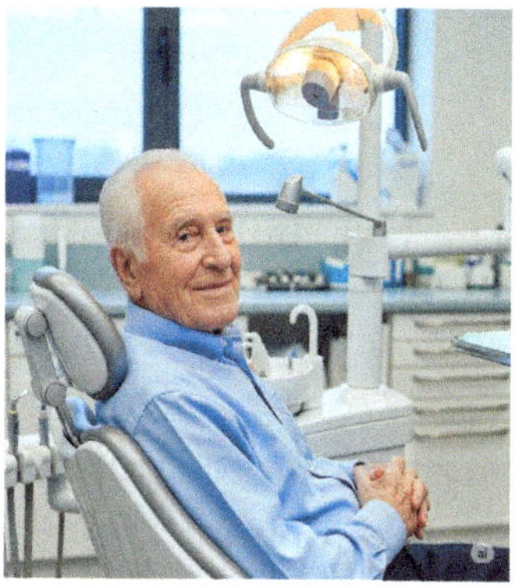

I shopped around and got three estimates. The first clinic want to remove a good molar to see if the wisdom tooth would recede back in the jaw line. If not then, charge me to remove the wisdom tooth. It is basically impossible to a tooth to recede, so this was a no-go decision

I then tried another clinic where they wanted a jaw dropping {like the pun?} $3,400.

I finally checked with my sister's dentist. He arranged for an oral surgeon who had to cut the wisdom tooth into 3 pieces to get it out. After I healed from the surgery, my primary dentist filled a few small cavities and did a thorough cleaning. Total costs: $1.100. Moral of the story? **It pays to shop.**

The dentist signed off that I was dentally cleared for transplant. That was the final box to check!

1.5 - Final Phone Check-In

My last step was a follow-up phone interview with the transplant team's social worker. They confirmed I had a support person to help me immediately after surgery. My insurance coverage was double-checked for any changes, and the dietitian made sure I understood some of the dietary changes I'd need to follow post-transplant.

After this phone call, I was placed on 'The List" but as pending / inactive.

I then waited for some lab draw kits to arrive from the transplant center. The schedule would be for me to take one kit a month - the first week of each month, to the dialysis clinic. The technician would draw the specified samples and ship them off overnight to U of M Hospital's lab.

Following the first blood sample being received and if no problems, I would be placed "Active". This was finally completed the last week in January, 2020.

Chapter 2 -Where Transplant Kidneys Come From

While this can be a long detailed subject to discuss, the high points are there are two options for kidney transplants. A third option – the bionic or mechanical is still being developed.

Here are the numbers of kidney transplants in the USA for the past five years:

- **2020:** 23,642 kidney transplants (including 5,234 from living donors and 18,408 from deceased donors).
- **2021:** 24,669 kidney transplants.
- **2022:** 25,498 kidney transplants.
- **2023:** 28,142 kidney transplants.
- **2024:** 27,759 kidney transplants.

I could not find any specific numbers but it is estimated between 25-30% of kidney transplants in the USA are from living donors, with the balance (70-75%) coming from deceased donors.

If you are trying to add those in your head, here is the total: 129,710. And note that March 2020 was the beginning of the COVID lock downs, or 2020 and maybe 2021 would have both been higher.

While organ buying, selling, and trading is strictly illegal in the United States, some other countries have different, more permissive laws or a laxer enforcement regarding organ donation and transplantation. This can result in the concept of "transplant tourism." U.S. citizens might be able to travel overseas to receive transplants, but they must be aware of the ethical and legal complexities. Not being a doctor or lawyer - I ain't touching this subject.

International bodies and conventions, like the Declaration of Istanbul, condemn organ trafficking and commercialism, urging countries to prohibit practices that exploit vulnerable populations. But it does happen, especially preying on vulnerable populations in the poorest of the poor areas of the world.

An overview summary of the process of matching and qualifying is discussed in more detail in

Chapter 3: Understanding Kidney Transplant List Placement

2.1 - Living Donors: The Gold Standard

Living donation is considered the gold standard of kidney transplants—for many reasons. While this could easily turn into a deep-dive discussion, I'll keep it brief.

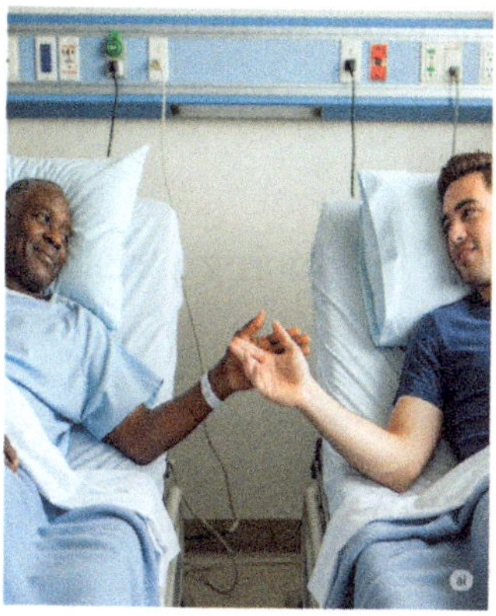

First and foremost: **The donor is generally not be responsible for any medical costs** related to the screening or the surgery. These expenses maybe covered by the transplant center or a third party. Neither the donor nor their insurance are commonly billed a dime for the transplant process itself.

However, things like lost wages, travel, hotel stays, meals, or parking fees *are not* covered by the transplant center. Those extra costs could be handled by the donor, the recipient, generous third parties, or even good fundraising efforts.

Another critical advantage is, unlike a deceased donation, the kidney is less shocked because the time from removal from the donor to placement in the recipient is much less.

2.1.1 - Why Living Donors Are Preferred

There are several advantages to receiving a kidney from a living donor:

- Longer transplant survival rates for the recipient
- Shorter wait times (no years-long national waiting list)
- Scheduled surgeries (no 2 a.m. "get to the hospital now" calls)
- Better donor-recipient matching, reducing risk of rejection

And here's something many people don't know:

A living donor doesn't have to be a family member or even someone you know. A complete stranger—moved by compassion, personal values, or just the desire to help—can step forward and donate.

If someone is feeling that kind of generosity, they can reach out to *any* hospital with a certified kidney transplant program and ask to speak with a transplant coordinator.

This is covered in the next section and also in Appendix 5 Being a Living Donor.

2.1.2 - Chains of Kindness

You might've heard of something called a **donor chain**. These are pretty incredible.

Say a family member wants to donate but isn't a match for their loved one. Instead, they donate to someone else on the waiting list who ***is*** a match. A loved one of that recipient pays it forward by entering the donor pool themselves. And so it continues.

Some of these chains have stretched across the country and helped dozens of people—all starting with one act of kindness. Although most chains are only a few donor/recipient pairs long, others are unimaginable.

Here are some of the longest Chains on record:

The 2012 National Kidney Registry Chain

- The longest chain at the time included **60 individuals** (30 donors and 30 recipients), spanning **17 hospitals across 11 U.S. states.**
- This chain was referred to as **Chain 124**, started by an altruistic donor (Rick Ruzzamenti) and lasted about four months

The 2014 Chain (70 Participants)

- In March 2015, the National Kidney Registry coordinated a chain of **70 participants**, breaking the previous record of 60
- This chain involved **35 transplants** across around 25 transplant centers, officially recognized by Guinness World Records

UAB Chain Surpassing 100

- The University of Alabama at Birmingham operated what became the **nation's longest single-site kidney transplant chain**, reaching over **100 living donors and recipients** by mid-2018.

UW Hospital's 34-Pair Chain (2015)

- At University of Wisconsin Hospital, a chain involving **34 donors and 34 recipients (68 individuals)** was completed, coordinated across 26 hospitals

2.2 - Deceased donors

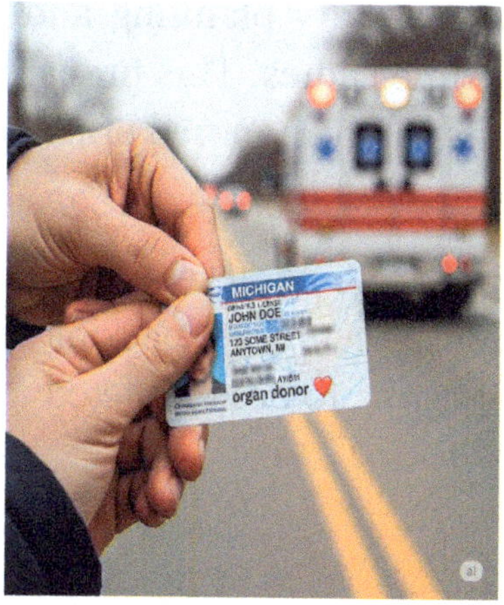

When it comes to organ transplantation, the most common source for kidneys and many other vital organs is a deceased donor. In the majority of these cases, the individual had made their wish to be an organ donor known prior to their death, often by registering their decision or indicating it on their driver's license.

However, during a medical emergency – the driver's license is seldom being checked by the treating medical teams. This is why it is important family / friends are aware so they may communicate the desires to the appropriate personnel at the hospital.

This deeply personal decision is one that should be openly discussed with close friends and family. While a formal registration is crucial, ensuring your loved ones are aware of your wishes can help simplify the process during a difficult time.

For organ donation to proceed, the treating medical team must be informed of the donor's desires **before death**, allowing for the necessary planning and scheduling of organ recovery when the time comes. This preparation ensures that the incredible gift of life can be honored efficiently and respectfully.

It may also be necessary to arrange for transportation from one medical center - possible in another state - for the organ harvesting to be completed properly.

2.3 -Bionic or Artificial Kidney

This is not currently an available option, but I am including a Addendum with more details on the status of these projects as of the writing of this book (Summer 2025).

Chapter 3 - Kidney Transplant List Placement

Some of this is boring and technical, feel free to skim it!!!!

3.1 - A Deep Dive into Allocation Factors

Alright, let's get one thing straight: This isn't the secret sauce recipe for getting a new kidney, nor is it the exhaustive, legal-text version of organ allocation. Think of it more as your "Cliffs Notes" or a friendly tour guide for the waiting list. We're hitting the highlights, not every single microscopic detail.

Being placed on the kidney transplant waiting list means you've been medically evaluated and deemed a suitable candidate for a new kidney.

The primary goals of the kidney allocation system are:

- **Maximize Graft Survival:** To ensure the donated kidney lasts as long as possible in the recipient.
- **Achieve Equity:** To distribute organs fairly among all qualified candidates.
- **Prioritize Medical Need & Urgency:** While recognizing chronic kidney disease is different from acute organ failure, certain medical circumstances do confer priority.

However, simply being "on the list" is just the first step.

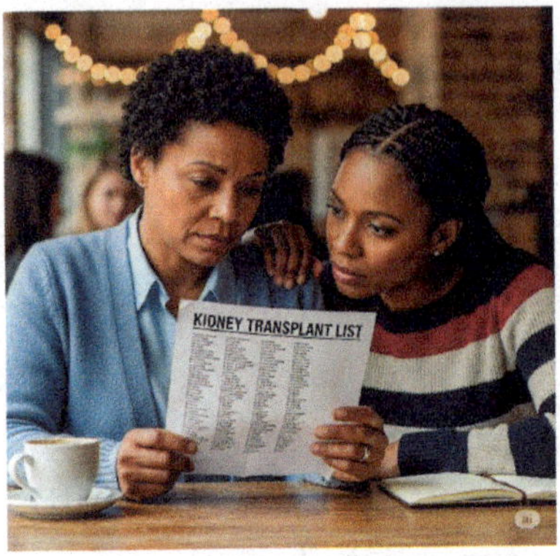

The actual process of matching a deceased donor kidney to a recipient is governed by a sophisticated system designed by the Organ Procurement and Transplantation Network (OPTN) and managed by the United Network for Organ Sharing (UNOS).

The OPTN/ UNOS system considers numerous factors to create a balanced approach to allocation.

3.2 - Medical Compatibility (The Non-Negotiables)

There are crucial biological matches required for a transplant to even be considered. Without compatibility, the recipient's immune system would rapidly and aggressively reject the new organ.

- **Blood Type (ABO Compatibility):** This is the most basic and absolute match. Just like a blood transfusion, donors and recipients must have compatible blood types

  One the most basic and important conditions are for Blood ABO cross matching and donor/recipient rules. e.g., Type A can receive from A or O; Type O can only receive from O. Of course there are additionally sub-sets such a O+, O-, A+, A-, etc. which may also be a factor.

- **HLA (Human Leukocyte Antigen) Matching:** HLAs are unique proteins found on the surface of most cells in the body, acting like a genetic fingerprint. The more HLA antigens the donor and recipient share, the better the "match," and generally, the lower the risk of the recipient's immune system attacking the new organ.

- **Body Size Match:** While not as life-or-death as blood and HLA compatibility, the size of the donor organ (especially for kidneys) should be appropriate for the recipient's body. This ensures proper anatomical fit within the abdominal cavity and optimal function once transplanted.

- **Crossmatch Test:** This crucial test is performed immediately before a transplant. It involves mixing the recipient's blood with the donor's white blood cells to see if the recipient has pre-formed antibodies that would immediately attack the donor's kidney. A "negative crossmatch" is absolutely essential – meaning no such antibodies are detected. A positive crossmatch indicates a high, immediate risk of hyperacute rejection, and the transplant would likely not proceed.

  This is one of the tests preformed with the blood drawn when you arrived at the transplant center.

3.3 - Medical Urgency & Desirability (Point System Drivers)

Beyond basic compatibility, several crucial factors influence your position on a kidney transplant waiting list. These elements are primarily integrated into a sophisticated point-based system designed to ensure fair and equitable allocation of organs.

3.3.1 - Age of Recipient and Donor: Age matters when matching kidneys. Usually, kidneys from older donors go to older recipients. Kidneys from younger donors—especially children—are often given to younger patients first. This helps the kidney last as long as possible in the person who gets it.

3.3.2 - Time on Dialysis: This is a major and highly impactful component of the Kidney Allocation System (KAS). Patients may accumulate valuable waiting time points from the date they begin dialysis or from the date they are medically approved for transplant. This acknowledges the profound burden and diminished quality of life associated with long-term dialysis, aiming to provide hope and a path forward for those who have been waiting the longest.

3.3.3 - Panel Reactive Antibody (PRA): Some patients have immune systems that are picky and react to many donor kidneys. This is called being "highly sensitized." It makes finding a match very hard. To help, these patients get extra priority on the transplant list so they still have a fair chance.

For example: if your PRA is 90%, it means your body would likely reject 90 out of 100 donor kidneys — only 10 might be a safe match.

3.3.4 - EPTS (Estimated Post-transplant Survival) and KDPI (Kidney Donor Profile Index): These are sophisticated predictive scores used in conjunction with age matching:

3.3.4.1 - EPTS: This score estimates how long a recipient is expected to live *after* a transplant, based on factors such as their age, the duration of their time on dialysis, any prior transplants, and the presence of diabetes. A lower EPTS score indicates a longer expected post-transplant survival.

3.3.4.2 - KDPI: Assesses the quality and expected longevity of a deceased donor kidney. It factors in donor characteristics like age, height, weight, ethnicity, cause of death, history of hypertension or diabetes, and creatinine levels. A lower KDPI indicates a higher quality kidney, generally expected to function for a longer period.

3.3.4.3 - How they interact: The allocation system aims to low KDPI kidneys with recipients having low EPTS. This strategy seeks to maximize the overall benefit and lifespan derived from each precious organ. However, it's important to note all kidneys are ultimately utilized; even kidneys with a higher KDPI can be successfully matched to recipients with a higher EPTS, providing significant life-enhancing benefits.

3.3.5 - Previous Transplant: If you've had a kidney transplant before, it can make finding a new match harder because your immune system may have built up more antibodies. But it doesn't mean you're off the waiting list. In fact, your past transplant or time already spent waiting might help boost your priority for a new one.

3.3.6 - Medical Stability and Suitability: To remain active on the waiting list, you must maintain medical stability. Active infections, active cancer, or significant deterioration in other vital organ systems could temporarily or even permanently suspend your listing. The transplant center continuously assesses your overall fitness for major surgery. Ensuring your body is ready to receive and sustain the new organ is paramount.

3.3.7 - Better Genetic Match Within the Same Ethnic Group: Kidney transplants work best when the donor and recipient share similar tissue types (like HLA markers). While matches can happen across races, people are more likely to match with someone of a similar ethnic background.

That means: Black, Hispanic/Latino, Asian, Native American, and other minority patients may wait longer for a match if fewer donors from their communities are registered.

3.3.7.1 - In the U.S., for example:

- White donors make up a larger portion of the donor registry.
- Black, Hispanic, Asian, and Native American communities are underrepresented, even though they make up a significant number of patients needing kidneys.

This can limit the pool of compatible organs for people in these groups.

3.3.7.2 - Living Donation: Ethnic Disparities Exist

Barriers to Living Donation can affect the available pool of both living and deceased donations.

- **Cultural & Religious Beliefs**

  Some cultures and faiths believe the body must remain whole after death or fear spiritual consequences. These beliefs can discourage both living and deceased donation.

- **Mistrust in Medicine**

  Historic mistreatment and bias have created deep mistrust in some minority communities. Potential donors may fear unfair treatment or exploitation by the medical system.

- **Lack of Awareness**

  Many are unaware living donation is an option. Misinformation about risks, recovery, and long-term health can also discourage potential donors.

- **The Power of Outreach**

  Culturally sensitive education led by trusted community voices can dispel myths, build trust, and encourage more people to consider living donation.

3.3.7.3 - Health Conditions Are Also a Factor

It's a really challenging situation that creates a double whammy. Certain health conditions like high blood pressure and diabetes are more common in some ethnic groups. These conditions can lead to kidney failure, which increases the number of people from those communities who desperately need a transplant.

Yet, those same health issues can make it harder to find a donor within their own family or community. Why? Because a potential living donor also needs to be in excellent health. If a family member also has high blood pressure or diabetes, they may not be healthy enough to donate a kidney safely.

So, while the need for transplants goes up, the healthy, willing donors who are a good match for that specific ethnic group can go down, making the wait even longer. It's a tough cycle that highlights why finding diverse donors is so important.

This is where the increase in affordable medical services can dull the knife on both sides –reducing the instances of kidney failure from untreated medical conditions while increasing the opportunities for donation (living and deceased) as there are more healthy donors available.

Increased education about the severity of this situation is also needed. Education at multiple levels including politicians, media influencers, community leaders, healthcare providers and the affected population groups.

Bottom Line

- Organs don't discriminate—but access to transplants and finding a compatible match can still be harder for some racial and ethnic groups.
- That's not because anyone's doing something wrong on purpose. It's often tied to things like unequal access to healthcare, different rates of certain diseases, and smaller donor pools in some communities.
- The more diverse our pool of organ donors, the better everyone's chances of finding the right match—regardless of background.
- These are tough but important conversations. Sharing stories - raising awareness - simply talking about donation in our families and communities can make a real difference.

3.4 - Geographic and Logistical Factors

Once medical compatibility and priority points are considered, the physical location of both the donor and recipient also plays a crucial role in organ allocation.

3.4.1 - Distance and Cold Ischemia Time: Kidneys, like all organs, have a limited "cold ischemia time"—the period they can be safely preserved outside the body before transplantation. To minimize this critical time and maximize the organ's viability, kidneys are offered first to recipients within the local donor service area (DSA).

If no suitable match is found locally, the organ is then offered regionally, and finally, if still unmatched, nationally. This tiered approach prioritizes efficiency and the best possible outcome for the transplanted organ.

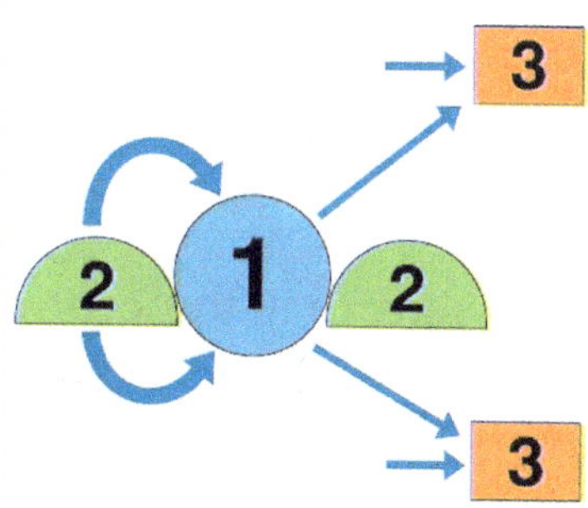

3.4.2 - Recipient Availability: When a compatible kidney becomes available, time is of the essence. The transplant center must be able to immediately contact the recipient and will start calling the provided list of contact numbers.

Once in contact with the recipient, after being briefed on the donation organ's history, the patient is asked if they want to accept or decline. Then, more importantly, can they arrive in specific time frame at the transplant center. Even if everything else aligns, if the patient is unable to arrive in time for surgery, the decision may be made to move on to the next on the list.

Unavailability for the transplant coordinator to reach the patient, even for a short period, could unfortunately lead to being passed over for that particular organ offer, as the team must move on to the next eligible candidate to preserve the organ's viability.

You should check with the transplant center for their policy on any affect being passed over because being unavailable will have on your list standing and placement.

When I signed up, to insure that the center could contact me where ever I was, I listed my cell phone number as primary, my Sister's as secondary, my two nieces as 3rd and 4th. The center would have called down the list and if unable to reach me or a representative – would have moved to the next candidate on the list.

3.5 – Declining an Offered Transplant

Let's say your phone rings—*the call* you've been waiting for. There's a kidney available, and you're next on the list. Exciting? Absolutely. But here's something not everyone realizes: you can actually decline that kidney.

Yes, really. Saying "no" to an offered transplant is a personal decision, and it happens. When you're offered an organ, you will receive basic information about the donor. This can include the donor's age, cause of death (like auto accident, stroke, trauma, or overdose), medical history, and how the organ has been preserved and transported.

Sometimes, the donor's background might raise flags. Maybe they had a health history that raises concerns for you. Or maybe the kidney itself has some unusual characteristics—perhaps it's from an older donor or someone with a higher-risk profile.

These factors don't automatically mean the kidney is "bad," but they can influence your comfort level.

So why might someone decline?

- **Medical reasons** – Maybe the kidney has a higher risk of delayed function or complications you're not prepared to accept.

- **Emotional readiness** – Some people just don't feel ready when the call comes. For example an external stress event like a sudden medical condition of a close loved one (even if not involved in your personal care)

- **Specific concerns** – You might want to wait for a donor closer in age, background, or health profile.

Here's the tricky part: declining an offer *may* affect your place on the transplant list. In some Donation Service Areas (DSAs), multiple declines could lead to a pause or review of your eligibility. In others, it may have no impact at all. This varies from region to region, and even from list to list within the same DSA.

Your transplant team will walk you through each offer and help weigh the pros and cons. Always ask questions, and remember: this is your life and your decision. It's not about being picky—it's about being informed and ready.

3.7 – Hitting the Pause Button

Sometimes life throws curve balls —an illness, insurance changes, issues regarding post-op care. When this happens, you can contact your transplant team to request to be placed on ***inactive*** status, also called pausing off the list.

This doesn't mean you're off the list or you will loose your spot. You simply aren't being considered for available organs while inactive. Your waiting time points *may* keep accumulating, and once you're reactivated, you're back in line.

Reasons for a pause can include:

- Medical issues that need to be resolved first (like an infection or heart concerns)
- Needing updated testing
- Travel or temporary life circumstances
- Insurance or financial coordination
- Your home care team having an issue and being unable to care for you if you receive your transplant.

It's nothing to be ashamed of, in fact, it can be a responsible choice—ensuring you're truly ready when that call comes. Every transplant center has its own policies, so be sure to ask how your center handles pauses and reactivations.

In closing

Your spot on the transplant waiting list isn't just a fixed number—it's part of a constantly moving equation. You're not competing against *everyone* on the list, only those who share key compatibilities with you, like blood type, organ size, and immune system match. As donor organs become available, a sophisticated points system compares candidates with similar profiles, factoring in things like medical urgency and time spent on dialysis. Your placement can shift as your condition changes or as others' circumstances evolve. While the process may seem mysterious at times, understanding how it works helps you advocate for yourself—and reminds you that this complex system is designed with one goal: to give everyone their best shot at a second chance.

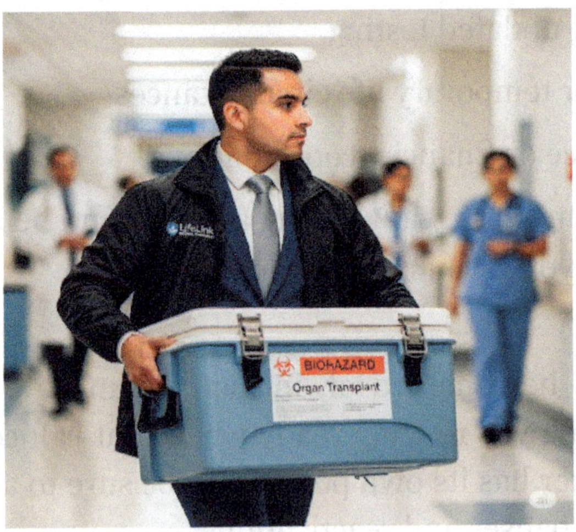

Chapter 4 - Double Listed: Multiple Transplant Lists

Being on Multiple Transplant Lists: Pros, Challenges, and Peace of Mind

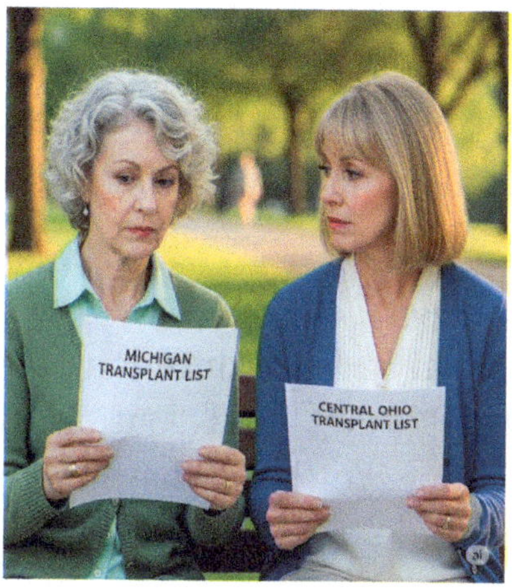

When you're fighting for your life, waiting on just one transplant list can feel like putting all your hope in one basket. That's why many patients explore **multiple listing**—registering at more than one transplant center to improve their chances of getting a kidney sooner.

It's not a loophole or a trick—it's a perfectly legal and often life-saving strategy recognized by the United Network for Organ Sharing (UNOS).

The biggest **advantage**? Geography matters. A lot. One transplant center might have an average wait time of 4–6 years. Another, just one state away, might only be 1–2 years. By listing in a different UNOS region—especially one with higher donor rates or fewer people on the wait list—you may dramatically shorten your wait. Example: California has two UNOS regions - north and south.

But like most things in life, there are a few speed bumps to plan for:

- *Every center has its own rules.* Being approved at one doesn't guarantee acceptance at another. You'll need to go through each center's evaluation process—sometimes in person, sometimes virtually.

- *Travel and logistics.* Getting to evaluation appointments, arranging lodging, and navigating follow-ups can be time-consuming and expensive.
- *Insurance can be a mixed bag.* Some plans support multiple listing (especially when it can reduce long-term dialysis costs), while others may limit out-of-state coverage or require more red tape. You might have trouble getting insurance to pay for out-of-state medications.

In my case, U of M Ann Arbor was the closest to us and it was a two hour drive each way - assuming no bad weather or traffic delays. Gas and time obligations add up quick - and much farther away might have also incurred motel expenses.

There's also the emotional side. Some patients wonder if it's fair to be on more than one list. Here's the thing: you're not jumping ahead of anyone. You're still only being considered when a kidney matches your specific compatibility criteria—blood type, antibody profile, size, and more. You're not competing against everyone on the list, just those you're medically matched with.

✓ **Bullet Points: Key Considerations**

- **What it means**: Being listed at more than one transplant center increases chances of getting a kidney.
- **Why do it**: Wait times vary by region—being listed in a different region might give you an edge.
- **Eligibility**: Each center will evaluate you; you must meet their all of requirements, including onsite testing.
- **Insurance**: Some insurance plans may cover multiple evaluations and listing.
- **Maintenance**: You must keep records updated, follow protocols at **each** center, and stay available in case a kidney becomes available.
- **Ethics and fairness**: Some critics say it favors people with more resources. Advocates say it's smart strategy if done transparently and ethically.
- **Living donation angle**: Being double-listed doesn't conflict with searching for a living donor—it expands your options. A living donor may be on the other listing wanting to give life without a matching patient.

Bottom line? This isn't about gaming the system. The transplant network is complex and ever-evolving. If multiple listing gives you a better shot at more time, more memories, and more life, then that's a route worth exploring. No guilt, just informed, proactive hope.

Chapter 5 - Legal Planning

Disclaimer: *Nothing in this chapter constitutes legal advice. Your personal circumstances are unique, and you must consult with properly licensed and trained professionals in your state of residence for tailored guidance. This information is intended solely to provide a foundational understanding, empowering you to ask informed questions of your legal and financial advisors.*

Most folks put off getting their legal papers in order because it means staring their own mortality right in the face—and that's not exactly a fun afternoon. They tell themselves there's plenty of time, so they keep kicking the can down the road. But ignoring those crucial legal and financial plans can leave family, loved ones, and beneficiaries in a real mess. In the end, a little preparation now can save a whole lot of heartache later.

5.1 - Plan today to ensure your wishes are honored

With over a decade as a Notary Public in Las Vegas, I frequently witnessed the critical consequences of delayed estate planning. All too often, I was called to hospitals and care facilities for critically ill individuals who had failed to plan.

For dialysis and transplant patients, proactive planning is even more crucial due to increased health risks. Anyone who has been on dialysis for very long has watched a patient transported out by EMS. Once, I was one of those people.

Major transitions—marriage, children, divorce, or even an unexpected inheritance—significantly impact your estate and highlight the need to review your plans. Modern blended families, in particular, underscore the importance of clearly defining inheritance chains to prevent disputes and uphold your intentions, especially concerning specific assets.

While numerous self-help resources provide valuable foundational information and basic forms, you must recognize their limitations. Estate planning isn't a "one-size-fits-all" endeavor. Fill in the blank forms may cause more issues than the solve. You can use these resources to grasp the fundamentals, but then consult with legal and financial professionals to create comprehensive documents tailored to your unique situation. Finally, re-check their advice against your research, and always ask questions.

The more thoroughly you plan and document your wishes , the more likely they will be respected by both your family and the courts. The following documents are essential considerations to discuss with your loved ones and competent advisors.

5.2 - Last Will and Testament

A "Will" offers clear instructions for asset distribution and guardianship, preventing family disputes and ensuring your wishes are honored. However, it typically requires a potentially lengthy and public probate process, and it only takes effect upon death, offering no provisions for incapacitation during life.

5.3 - Trusts

Trusts avoid probate, allowing faster asset distribution and greater control than wills. They can also manage assets long-term, but are costlier, complex, and must be properly funded with legal help—*not!!!* a DIY task

Trusts are not hard you say? You read some posts online, you watched a few videos. A website offered easy trusts, just answer some questions and download the final documents Easy right?

Do you know the difference between a straight trust and an A-B Trust? When should you use an A-B-C trust? Can you describe A QTIP Trust and when to best use it? Revocable vs Non-Revocable? Can you - and should you - have multiple trusts for different assets and beneficiaries? How do you move assets into or out of a trust? Tax implications??

I only brushed there are the differences in trusts. Get a lawyer, please?

5.4 - Wills vs Trusts

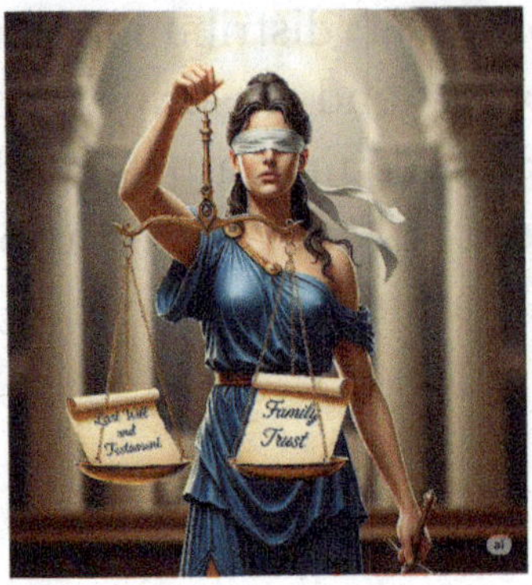

Wills are generally simpler and less expensive to create, primarily directing asset distribution and naming guardians for minors after death, but they typically require a public, lengthy and costly probate court process.

Trusts, while more complex and costly to establish, offer privacy, avoid probate, and can manage assets both during life and after death, providing greater control over how and when beneficiaries receive their inheritance. Often, a comprehensive estate plan will strategically utilize both wills and trusts to maximize benefits.

5.5 - Advance Directive

An Advance Directive is a legal document that articulates your healthcare wishes if you become unable to make decisions for yourself. Who can make decisions for you and your preferences for medical treatments, life support. It's main benefit is ensuring your autonomy and relieving loved ones of difficult choices during a crisis and promoting peace of mind. However, these documents require careful consideration, clear communication with your designated healthcare agent, and periodic updates to reflect changing wishes or medical advancements.

5.6 - Living Will

A Living Will is a specific type of Advance Directive that outlines your preferences for life-sustaining medical treatments, such as ventilators or feeding tubes, what to do if you are terminally ill or in a permanently unconscious state and unable to communicate. Its primary benefit is providing clear instructions for end-of-life care, ensuring your wishes are honored and alleviating difficult decisions for your family.

However, a living will only applies in very specific medical scenarios and may not cover all unforeseen situations, emphasizing the importance of also designating a healthcare agent.

5.7 - Durable Power of Attorney for Healthcare (DPOA-HC) / Healthcare Proxy / Medical Power of Attorney

This document designates a trusted individual, your "healthcare agent" or "proxy," to make medical decisions on your behalf if you become unable to communicate. Unlike a Living Will, which outlines specific treatments, the DPOA-HC empowers your chosen agent to interpret your values and make decisions across a broader range of medical situations, including unforeseen circumstances. This provides flexibility and ensures someone you trust can advocate for you when you cannot.

5.8 - Do Not Resuscitate (DNR) Order

A DNR order is a medical order that specifically instructs healthcare providers *not* to perform cardiopulmonary resuscitation (CPR) if your heart stops or you stop breathing. While your wishes regarding CPR might be mentioned in a Living Will, a separate DNR is a direct, actionable medical order that is immediately accessible to emergency personnel. It ensures your specific desire to avoid resuscitation is clearly documented and respected, preventing unwanted interventions.

5.9 - Physician Orders for Life-Sustaining Treatment (POLST) / Medical Orders for Life-Sustaining Treatment (MOLST)

These are medical orders created in consultation with your physician for individuals who are seriously ill or near the end of life. They translate your advance directive wishes into actionable medical orders that are followed immediately by all healthcare providers, including EMS. POLST/MOLST forms are designed to be portable, universally recognized, providing clear guidance on specific treatments like resuscitation, intubation, and feeding tubes. They effectively bridge the gap between your legal wishes and immediate medical care.

5.10 - Organ Donation Authorization

Organ Donation Authorization is your legal consent to donate organs, eyes, and tissues after death, usually noted on your driver's license or in a state registry. It offers the "gift of life," helping multiple people and bringing comfort to loved ones. Most religions support donation, and it won't prevent traditional funeral arrangements. Be sure to share your decision with family, as some states may still request their consent.

Yes, in case you are curious - I am a Registered Organ Donor. I was before I needed one, and I remain on the list. Being an organ Donor is a personal decision and not everyone is comfortable doing it. Which is fine.

5.11 - Funeral Arrangements / Letter of Instructions

A Letter of Instructions (also known as a Letter of Last Instruction or Final Wishes Letter) is an informal, non-legally binding document.

This letter provides details on everything from desired funeral or memorial preferences to obituary information to the location of important documents. It may list accounts, and digital logins, easing the administrative burden on your family.

Though not necessarily legally enforceable, its immense value lies in offering clarity, reducing disputes over personal effects, and providing peace of mind by clearly communicating your final wishes. Seems simple but lawyer review is still recommended.

5.11.1 - Prepaid Funeral Home Plans

Pre-arranged/Pre-paid funeral plans can legally lock in specific services and costs with a funeral home. Research these carefully as they are not always a good financial investment because of their strict lock in of services and service providers.

5.12 - Internment of your remains

Interment is the burial or placement of remains in a permanent site, like a cemetery or columbarium.

5.12.1 - Burial Plot

The burial plot with a head stone/marker is the most well know and traditionally recognized. It is also the most expensive. With our modern mobile society, families may be far flung across the USA or even the world. Getting an agreement on where the burial plot will be physically could be contentious among family members. Whether they are fighting to have you closer to them or farther away, is not a conversation I am going to get involved in. But either way, if you have a preference, you might want to include it in your Letter of Instruction.

5.12.2 - Columbarium

A columbarium (for cremated) is less expensive – but also less personal as it may look like a locker wall in a bus station with dozens or even 100s all together.

See Burial plot for discussion on where it should be located.

5.12.3 - National Cemeteries - Veterans Affairs

Veterans often receive either a burial plot or a columbarium. These will include a marker and may/may not include Full Military Honors.

5.13- Cremation vs. Burial

Cremation offers flexibility in memorialization and can be more environmentally conscious, often at a lower immediate cost than a traditional burial. However, it's an irreversible process, and crucially, in many states (including Michigan), the legal next-of-kin must provide authorization *even if* the deceased expressed a wish for cremation in their will. Burial offers a permanent resting place for visits and traditional mourning, aligning with many cultural and religious practices. Though often more costly due to plot, casket, and service fees, it provides a physical space for remembrance.

5.14 - Named Funeral Representative

In some states, like Michigan, you can legally designate a "Named Funeral Representative" to make decisions about your funeral and the disposition of your remains, overriding the default next-of-kin hierarchy (spouse, children, etc.). This provides crucial control, ensuring your specific wishes are honored, especially if family dynamics are complex or your closest confidant isn't a legal relative. While it offers peace of mind and can prevent family disputes, this designation must be properly documented and typically requires the representative's acceptance, highlighting the importance of clear communication and careful planning. Check with your specific state and be aware that the laws can and do change so it may be necessary to update to reflect recent changes. Michigan last changed it's law in 2016.

5.15 - Power of Attorney: Because Life Doesn't Pause for Paperwork

We have reviewed many different documents. But most are singular purpose, limited scope. And if nothing else, life is seldom straightforward and one sided. For those situations you need more power and flexibility. Enter: the Power of Attorney (POA)—basically the legal version of tagging someone **"it"** when life body-slams you.

5.15.1 - What is a Power of Attorney

A Power of Attorney lets someone else handle your business when you can't. This could mean writing checks, selling a car, wrangling with your insurance company, or making sure your dog gets his monthly BarkBox. Okay, maybe not that last one. But the rest? Totally fair game.

5.15.2 - One Size Fits All? Nope

POAs can be broad (think: "You can do pretty much anything I could do") or specific ("You're only allowed to sell my house, not touch my vintage vinyl collection"). The beauty is, you're the boss. You get to decide who does what, and how much power they have, when the power starts and stop as well as you can revoke it at will.

5.15.3 - Why It Matters

During transplant time, you may be out of commission. Not permanently—but long enough that someone may need to sign, sell, pay, or organize on your behalf. You need the right people with the paperwork and the authority to act on your behalf. Fewer panicked phone calls and no "Oops, your mortgage is late" surprises.

5.15.4 - Yes, you can have more than one flavor

In fact, it's kind of like building your own legal Justice League:

- Put your daughter in charge of real estate—she's great with Zillow and elbow grease.

- Give your financial-savvy buddy access to your investments—he lives for spreadsheets.

- Maybe your cousin handles the bills—she already balances three kids, two dogs, and a side hustle. She can juggle a few utility payments.

- If you have children or other dependents, you might want to have the person(s) who are overseeing any trusts / investments / assets to be different than the person(s) who are caring for them.

5.15.5 - Pro tips before you hand over the keys:

- Trust is key. Make sure the people you choose are responsible, reliable, and not likely to disappear to Mexico with your savings. Or your dog.
- Be clear. Spell out what powers each person has in detail. If only one person is allowed to drive your 1976 Candy Apple Red White Convertible Top Ford Mustang, put it in writing. Vague POAs are a lawyer's retirement plan.
- Put it in writing. Use a reputable legal service or talk to an estate attorney in your state. A cocktail napkin and good intentions won't cut it in court, even if the bartender and a waitress signed as witnesses.

Bottom line: Power of Attorney doesn't mean you've given up control—it just means you're smart enough to share the load *before* things hit the fan.

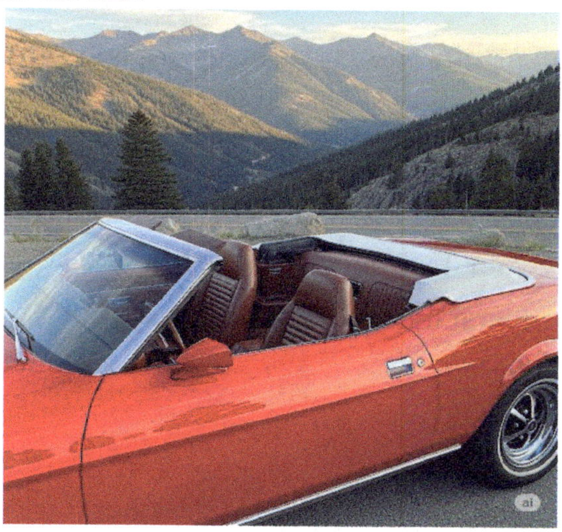

5.16 - Notary Public - the nuts and bolts

You will notice that some of the documents thus far discussed require a notary. You've probably had something notarized at some point—a will, a power of attorney, maybe even a car title—but did anyone *ever* explain what the notary was actually doing, aside from stamping your paperwork like it was a coffee shop loyalty card?

5.16.1 - What the heck is a Notary Public

A Notary Public is a state-appointed official whose job is to help prevent fraud. <u>That's it in a nutshell.</u> They don't give legal advice. They <u>won't</u> give legal advice. They don't write your documents for you or tell you how to complete fill-in-the-blank forms and (contrary to popular belief) they don't "make it legal."

Your document *already* carries legal weight—the notary is just there to confirm a few critical things:

- You are who you say you are
- You're signing willingly (not under duress or threats of losing your TV remote)
- You understand what you're signing

5.16.2 - What Notaries Do:

- Check ID (not your library card—actual government-issued ID)
- Witness signatures
- Administer oaths or affirmations
- Fill out and attach a notarial certificate (wordy little phrases like "subscribed and sworn before me...")

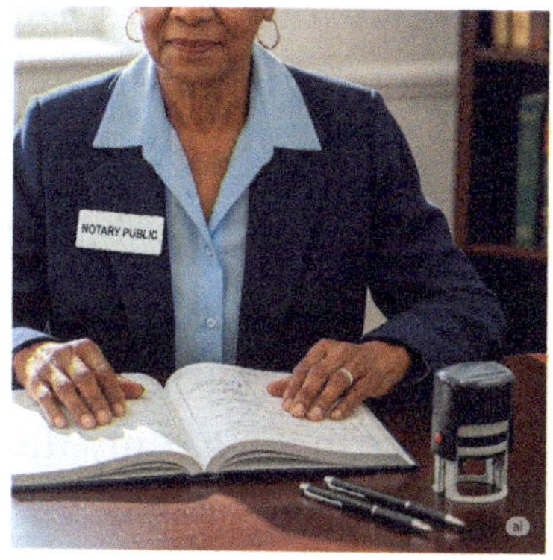

The notary will a fix their seal (ink stamp, embossed or both), sign an existing Notary Statement on the document or attach a separate one and sign their signature.

They will also add your information to their log book including the type of ID used and information from it, plus your name and address and have you sign the book.

They may or may not also take a thumb or finger print. Few do this but some do, especially common with real estate documents.

That's it. No law degrees, no Jedi mind tricks, just verification, impartiality, and a trusty journal and stamp.

5.16.3 - What Notaries don't:

- Give legal advice (Nope. Not even a little!).
- Tell you which form to use (That's a job for a lawyer, not your neighborhood notary).
- Explain how to fill out the forms you downloaded from some DIY legal advise website. (Again, you need a lawyer with training, knowledge and expertise.)
- Make copies into "certified" copies of things like birth certificates (only the states do this). Other documents like marriage licenses or adoption certificates might also be restricted for a notary to 'certify' a copy. If they say 'No, I can not do that' - please don't get mad, they are fallowing the laws of the state.
- Use invisible ink or seal things with wax.
- Certify pinky swears.

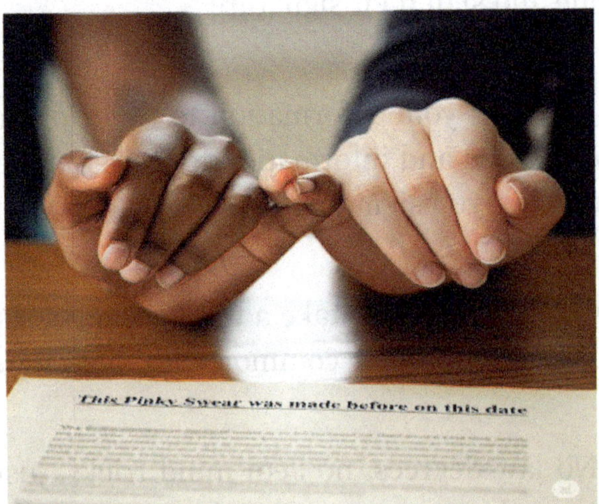

5.16.4 - Where To Find A Notary Public

You can find notaries in a variety of places, but not all notaries are available to the general public, even if the name says public in it. This restriction is often related to their employment.

For example, many banks have notaries on staff, but they may only provide services to their customers — and sometimes only for bank-related documents.

Other notaries work at businesses like mail and shipping stores (e.g., UPS Stores, Postal Annex), which often offer walk-in notary services.

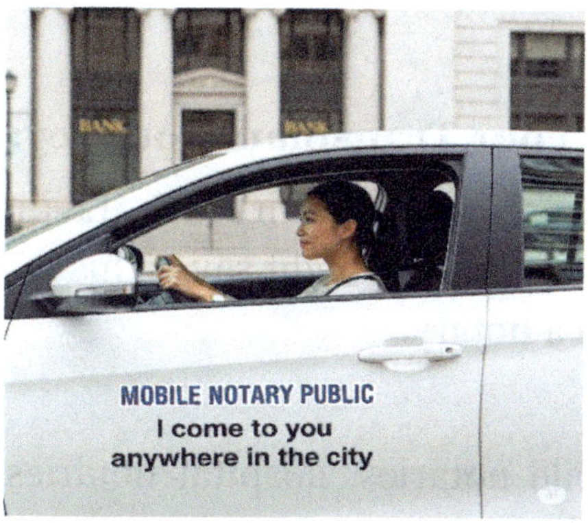
BANK
BANK
MOBILE NOTARY PUBLIC
I come to you
anywhere in the city

You'll also find **mobile notaries** who will come to your home, office, or even meet you at a local café or diner. If you know a **real estate agent or mortgage broker**, they often work with notaries regularly and can refer someone reliable

A quick online search for **"mobile notary public near me"** will bring up local listings.

5.16.5 - Pro Tip: Ask Before You Book

If you're calling based on an online search, explain:

- What you need notarized
- How many documents
- How many people will sign

Then ask for their fees, and be sure to call at least two for comparison.

While some states regulate notary fees strictly, others do not — and frankly, some notaries get a little "creative" with how they calculate their total cost, especially for mobile services. It pays to ask questions upfront.

5.16.6 - Why This Matters for Your Transplant Journey:

If you're signing a Power of Attorney, Advance Directive, Living Will, or any other document where someone might say, "This is a big deal," chances are—you'll need a notary.

And during a health crisis? Mobile notaries, hospital notaries, and even remote online notaries (in some states) can step in and help. But don't wait until the last second while hooked up to a heart monitor. Getting your documents signed and notarized ahead of time gives you peace of mind—and your loved ones fewer headaches.

In Closing, Don't Wait For Legal Planning

While this chapter focuses on transplant-specific concerns, the documents and guidance apply to everyone — young or old, sick or healthy, single or married, with dependents (people kids or pet-kids) or flying solo.

In my younger days as a notary, I was often called to hospital rooms and care facilities to assist with emergency documents. Once, to the heartbreak of family — I could not validate the cognitive abilities of the signer. *Don't be that person.*

Another notary might have proceeded, but I personally refused because I wasn't convinced the gentleman understood the gravity of the paperwork in front of him — or even had the ability to sign his name independently. *Don't wait until it's too late.* Make your decisions with a clear head and sound conscience. It bears repeating: *people don't plan to fail — they fail to plan.*

Chapter 6 - Insurance and Financial

A Vital Note: Rules Change!

What worked for me back in 2019/2020 in Michigan probably will not apply to you—every state and program changes on the regular. Think of this guide as your friendly roadmap, but your transplant social worker and financial coordinator? They're your real MVPs. They know the latest rules and programs and should be your go-to for any specific questions.

If you're facing or experiencing kidney failure, a transplant can feel like hitting the reset button on life. But let's be honest—handling the medical stuff is just half the battle. The money side, especially insurance, often makes or breaks whether you get the green light as a candidate.

Transplant centers have to follow tight financial rules—not to make things tricky, but because it takes more than a surgery to make it work. There's meds, labs, checkups - for life. They want to be sure you can handle that road ahead.

This chapter gives you the basics on insurance and what to expect money-wise. Policies and programs change by place, but this should help you learn about things you need to ask about.

6.1 - Why Insurance Coverage is Non-Negotiable

(The "Why" Behind the Financial Requirements)

A kidney transplant isn't a one-time event — it's a lifelong commitment to medical care. That's why insurance coverage isn't just preferred; it's required. Transplant centers aren't being overly cautious or cold. They have to ensure that both the organ and the recipient have the best chance of long-term success. Here's why insurance matters so much:

6.1.1 - Astronomical Costs Go Beyond Surgery

The transplant process includes far more than just the operation itself. Patients must go through extensive pre-transplant evaluations (labs, scans, specialist consults), organ acquisition costs, the actual surgery, plus hospital stays and initial in-clinic follow ups.. This adds up quickly — and that's before the ongoing costs begin.

One example of the on going costs to the transplant center is the monitoring of lab reports. Every time you go in for your monthly or bi-monthly lab reports, the results are sent to the transplant center for your transplant nephrologist to review and adjust your medications if needed.

6.1.2 - Anti-Rejection Medications Are Expensive and Lifelong

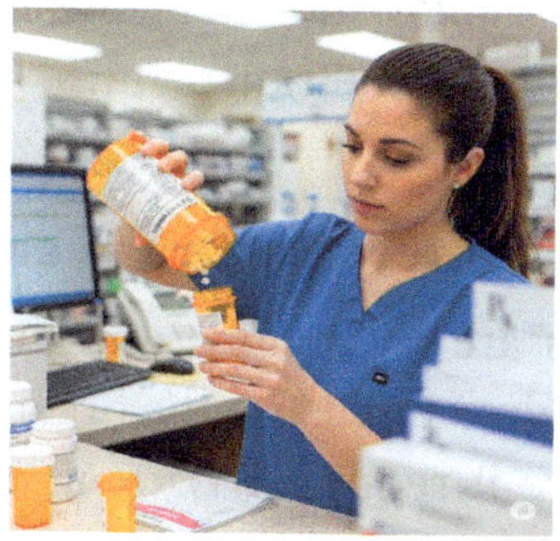

Immunosuppressants must be taken every single day, for life. These drugs are not optional – they are the bodyguard for your new kidney. Without insurance, monthly costs can easily reach into the thousands. If a patient can't afford these meds, the organ is at risk of rejection.

If you lose coverage unexpectedly, many hospitals have access to emergency assistance programs for high-cost medications. This is why it's vital to stay in regular contact with your transplant center's social workers. They're often the first to hear about new insurance options and financial aid programs—sometimes before they're widely announced.

One of my required medications retails for over $1,000 a month. For many, choosing the right insurance isn't just paperwork—it's the difference between affording food and housing, **or** life-saving medicine.

6.1.3 - Monitoring & Follow-Ups Never End

After a transplant, patients must undergo frequent lab testing, clinic visits, and sometimes readmission to the hospital. This level of follow-up is medically necessary, and any lapse can compromise the transplant.

6.1.4 - Protect the Organ and the Patient

Organs are a precious and limited resource. Transplant teams have a duty to ensure the organ goes to someone who can sustain the care it requires. Without access to regular medications and care, a patient is at high risk of graft failure and serious complications.

6.1.5 - Avoiding Financial Ruin

Even with insurance, transplant-related costs can be overwhelming. Without it, the financial burden can be devastating. Transplant centers don't want patients to end up drowning in debt that could affect their ability to stay healthy.

6.1.6 - Program Sustainability

Transplant programs are costly to run and heavily regulated. Hospitals need to be reimbursed for the complex care they provide. Financial stability on both ends — the patient and the provider — is essential to keep these programs running for future patients.

6.2 - The "Two-Source" Requirement:

During my own transplant evaluation, I was required to have at least two independent sources of insurance coverage. This isn't unique to me—it's a common requirement across many transplant centers nationwide. This strategy isn't meant to create unnecessary red tape; it's a practical and protective measure with several important goals:

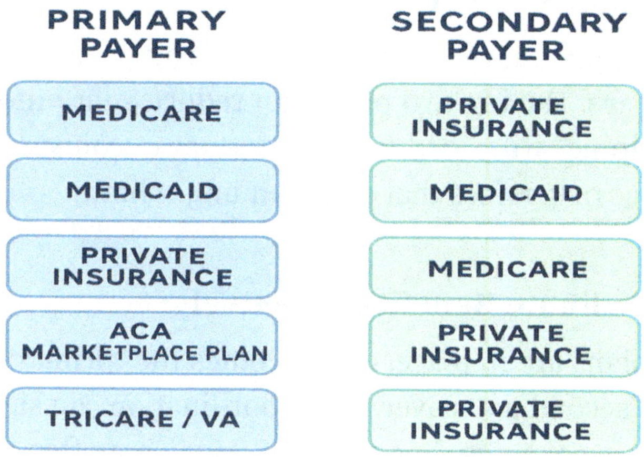

Note: This is a SAMPLE chart only.

Medicaid could act as a primary or secondary payer, depending on whether the patient's other insurance. If no other coverage exists, Medicaid is primary. If paired with Medicare or private insurance, it typically acts as secondary—covering eligible costs not paid by the primary plan. Even with multi-plans, you may still have co-pays you are responsible for paying.

6.2.1 - Provide a Safety Net:

If one insurance plan changes, is canceled, or becomes less comprehensive—as often happens with job changes, aging out of coverage, or policy revisions—the second plan can act as a backup. This helps ensure there is no interruption in coverage for critical, ongoing care.

6.2.2 - Maximize Coverage:

Even strong insurance plans may not cover every aspect of transplant care. Having two plans can reduce your out-of-pocket burden, helping with deductibles, co-pays, coinsurance, and specific drugs or services that one plan might limit.

6.2.3 - Coordinate Benefits Effectively:

When two plans are in place, one becomes the "primary" and the other the a "secondary" payer. This coordination can significantly reduce gaps in coverage. For example, Medicare often acts as the primary insurer, while a secondary private or employer-based plan may cover the remainder—this is especially important with high-cost medications and services.

6.3 - Common Types of Insurance Coverage for Transplant Candidates:

Transplant centers generally accept a combination of the following insurance types. Each comes with its own rules, benefits, and limitations—understanding these is essential to meeting eligibility requirements and ensuring long-term care.

6.3.1 - Medicare

ESRD Eligibility: Individuals diagnosed with End-Stage Renal Disease (ESRD) typically become eligible for Medicare (Parts A and B) after a short waiting period—often three months after starting dialysis or immediately after receiving a transplant.

6.3.1.1 - What It Covers:

Part A: Inpatient hospital care

Part B: Outpatient care and physician services

Part D: Prescription drugs, including immunosuppressants

6.3.1.2 - Medicare 36-Month Cliff:

- Part A (Hospital Insurance): Your coverage for inpatient hospital care, skilled nursing facilities, and other services under Part A ends 36 months after the month of your successful kidney transplant.

- Part B (Medical Insurance): Your coverage for doctor visits, outpatient services, and other medical supplies also terminates at the 36-month mark.

  However, there is a crucial exception that was recently enacted. As of January 1, 2023, a new benefit called the Part B-Immunosuppressive Drug Benefit (Part B-ID) was created. This benefit allows individuals in this exact situation to enroll in a limited form of Part B that covers only immunosuppressive drugs for the rest of their lives.

- Part D (Prescription Drug Coverage): If you had a Part D plan, your coverage for all other medications (besides the immunosuppressive drugs covered by the Part B-ID benefit) ends along with your Part A and Part B coverage at the 36-month mark.

This limitation is one of the primary reasons why a secondary insurance source is so often required.

6.3.1.3 - What happens when you fall off the cliff

The "cliff" is a combination of your Part A and full Part B coverage ending. While the new Part B-ID benefit provides a critical safety net for immunosuppressive drugs, it is not a substitute for comprehensive health coverage.

You would be responsible for finding other insurance to cover all other medical needs, including lab tests, doctor visits, and non-immunosuppressive medications, unless or until you re-qualify for Medicare due to age or disability.

A simple reason for the cut off of Medicare after 36 months is the belief that once you are off of dialysis - unless otherwise disabled - you can return to the work force and provide your own insurance via your employer or the ACA Marketplace.

6.3.2 - Medicaid

State-Dependent Program: Medicaid is jointly funded by federal and state governments but administered by each state, meaning transplant-related coverage varies widely. Potential Role:

- In some states, Medicaid serves as a primary payer; in others, it functions as secondary, helping to cover gaps left by Medicare or private insurance.
- However, Medicaid may limit provider options or services, making coordination with your transplant center essential.

6.3.3 - Employer-Sponsored

You have employer group sponsored insurance from a private company, a government agency, a union or other group plan. The coverage available for transplant vary vastly in these plans and are subject to change. Contact your plan administer for details.

6.3.4 - ACA Marketplace Plans

(Affordable Care Act)

Viable Option: ACA plans may serve as either primary or secondary insurance. They can be especially helpful for those without employer-sponsored insurance.

Important Considerations:

- Ensure your transplant center is listed as in-network.
- Review the **formulary** (covered drugs list) to confirm coverage of **immunosuppressants**.
- Understand cost-sharing and out-of-pocket maximums.
- Check for lifetime maximums. Although ACA forced some companies to remove limits from policies - a great plan could have limits on specific items that might haunt you in the future.

6.3.5 - Military Health Coverage (TriCare, VA Benefits)

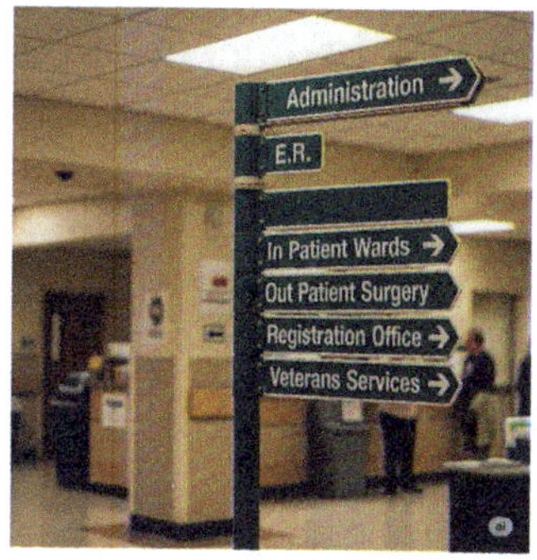

Who Qualifies: Active duty military, veterans, retirees, and their dependents.

- **Coverage**: These programs may generally offer robust transplant coverage, often with fewer out-of-pocket costs than civilian plans.
- **Caveats**:
    - Must comply with the **referral process** and care coordination systems required by TRICARE or the VA.
    - Check that your transplant center accepts these benefits and can bill them properly.

One major problem with some VA/TriCare benefits can be the lack of available hospitals or clinics close to you.

I have also personally had problems in the past getting prescriptions approved thru the VA hospital. I have heard it has improved, but I have not re-checked because I was able to secure other insurance to handle it. If you qualify - there is no reason to not ask.

6.4 - What to Look for in a Policy

When evaluating insurance options for transplant, don't stop at checking for "transplant coverage." Check critical areas:

- Out-of-Pocket Maximums: What is the maximum you'll be responsible for paying annually or lifetime? This cap can be a lifesaver when costs soar.
- Deductibles and Coinsurance: How much must you pay before your insurance kicks in, and what portion are you responsible for after that?
- Medication Coverage — Especially Anti-rejection: This is vital. Review the drug formulary, tiers, and any annual or lifetime limits.
- Network of Providers: Is the transplant center and its affiliated surgeons, specialists, and hospitals in network? Out-of-network care can be financially devastating.
- Travel and Lodging Assistance: Some centers are far from home. While rare, certain plans or assistance programs may cover some travel or lodging during evaluation, surgery, or follow-up.
- Rehabilitation and Support Services: Does the policy cover post-transplant services such as:
    - Physical therapy?
    - Mental health care?
    - Nutritional counseling?

Each of these can be essential for recovery and long-term health. But broken record – each person and their needs will vary.

Pro Tip

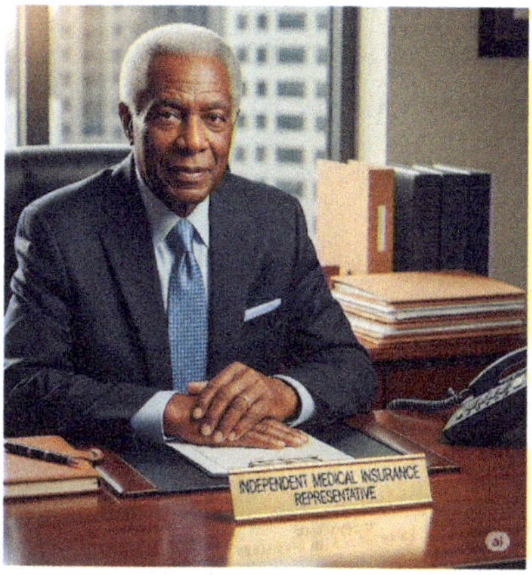

Independent agents work with multiple companies, so they can help you mix and match coverage—like health insurance from one, prescriptions from another, and vision or dental from a third. They use their experience to find the best overall coverage and value—not just the cheapest premium.

The implementation of the Affordable Care Act (ACA) and launch of the HealthCare Marketplace (https://www.healthcare.gov/) made coverage accessible for millions of people who previously couldn't afford it.

But while the site offers useful tools, choosing the right plan can still be confusing. That's why I recommend working with an independent health insurance agent. They stare at those plans all day long and understand the ins-and-outs of the plans - matching you to the one that closest matches your needs.

6.5 -The Role of the Transplant Financial Coordinator

Every transplant center employs a **financial coordinator**—and they're one of your most important allies in this process.

Here's what they do:

- Verify Coverage
  They'll evaluate your current insurance to confirm it meets transplant center requirements.

- Identify Gaps
  They're trained to spot weak points—whether that's limited drug coverage or inadequate secondary insurance.

- Maybe Help with Applications
  From Medicare and Medicaid to grant or foundation support, they may be able guide you through applying for coverage you might not know you qualify for.

Tip: Stay in regular contact with your coordinator. Policies and financial criteria can change. They'll help you stay compliant and covered.

6.6 - What If You're Uninsured or Underinsured?

If you don't have insurance—or your current coverage isn't enough—don't panic. You're not out of options. Many people in your situation have successfully navigated transplant with the right help and persistence.

Patience <u>and</u> Persistence. It took you many times to learn to tie your shoes but you persisted and prevailed. Don't let one NO or Not Qualified stop you from your goal of getting a transplant.

Here's what to know and where to start:

6.6.1 - Talk to the Your Financial Coordinator Immediately

They've seen every type of insurance situation imaginable. Their job is to:

- Help you explore every possible source of coverage
- Connect you with programs and emergency resources
- Determine if your state Medicaid or a transplant-specific grant could help

6.6.2 - Medicaid Might Be an Option (Even if You Think You Don't Qualify)

Medicaid eligibility varies by state, changes often, and transplant-related needs can sometimes open doors that weren't previously available.

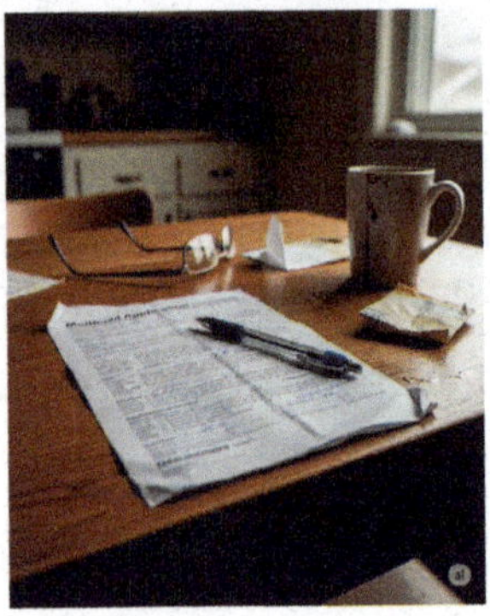

Some people may qualify due to:

- Income and asset changes during medical leave
- Disability status
- Spending down to meet Medicaid thresholds ("Medically Needy" programs)

A financial coordinator or local Medicaid specialist can guide you through the application process.

6.6.3 - Apply for Medicare if You're Eligible

If you have end-stage renal disease (ESRD) or another qualifying condition, you may be eligible for **Medicare**, even if you're under 65. In many cases:

- Medicare kicks in retroactively
- It can work alongside Medicaid or a secondary plan
- You may need both Parts A & B, and likely Part D for prescriptions

6.6.4 - Look Into Marketplace Plans or State Exchanges

If you're uninsured and not yet eligible for Medicare/Medicaid, the Affordable Care Act (ACA) marketplace may offer a plan that:

- Covers transplant services and medications
- Comes with subsidies or reduced premiums based on your income

You may also qualify for a *Special Enrollment Period* due to major health or financial changes.

6.6.5 - Seek Help from Foundations and Grant Programs

Several organizations help transplant patients bridge financial gaps for medications, transportation, housing, and even premiums. Examples include:

- National Foundation for Transplants
- American Transplant Foundation
- Local nonprofit transplant assistance programs

6.6.6 - Fundraising is More Common Than You Think

Many patients turn to community fundraising platforms (like GoFundMe) or work with groups like Help Hope Live, which help set up tax-deductible medical fundraising pages and provide tools to track expenses. Chapter 7 Hope with Honor: Raising Funds Without Losing Dignity covers this in more details.

Wrapping It Up:

The Insurance Part Isn't the Wall—It's the Door

If insurance talk has your head spinning, take a breath. You've just absorbed a crash course in something most people never expect to learn—but *you're still standing*. That says a lot. Yes, it's complicated. HMO, PPO, ESRD, CMS... cue the eye-roll. You don't have to know it all. You just have to ask the questions.

Every year, people with every kind of insurance situation—good, bad, and nonexistent—get listed for transplant. Start checking all your options: Medicaid, Medicare, private plans, foundations, grants, exchanges, fundraising, VA, union, railroad, or government retiree benefits. So yes, it takes research. But it's doable. And once you've got the right coverage, the road ahead can feel a lot smoother.

When I hit the Medicare Cliff, I was comparing plans and looking at the cost of the monthly premiums. Being confused I charted the premiums and co-pays for expensive and cheaper plans.

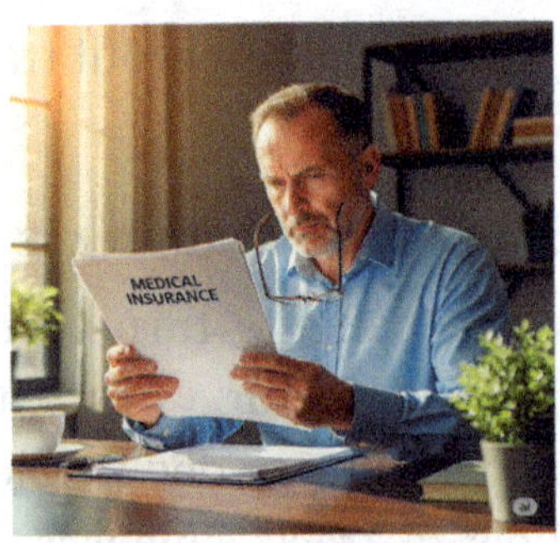

I discovered a more expensive premium plan actually cheaper because it covered more of my medications with lower co-pays.

Chapter 7 - Raising Funds Without Losing Dignity

You don't lose dignity by asking for help.
You lose it pretending you never needed any.

This chapter is about showing you how to:

- Ask with grace
- Receive with dignity
- And give others the opportunity to help you live
- Importance of being upfront and honest. Always.
- More ways than you could have imiganed to receive support

Sadly, too many of us have offered money, groceries, or a ride to someone—only to discover they didn't need it, they just wanted it for free. We've seen the headlines: phony charities, fundraisers where 90% of donations landed in someone's pocket but the actual cause, and the kind of scams that make everyone more hesitant to give.

But you're not a scam. You're someone facing a real-life medical crisis. And handled the right way, your fundraising will be rooted in integrity, clarity, and hope. It will be genuine, honest and effective.

So now, let's take a walk—arm in arm with honesty and humility—down the yellow brick road to the pot of gold at the end of the rainbow. Maybe not a pot of atomic number 79 but what you need to cover your gas, meds, and maybe a burrito.

7.1 - No one plans to need a kidney transplant.

And no one plans for the cost that comes with it. Not just the surgery, but travel, time off work, post-op medications, and the life adjustments that ripple far beyond your hospital stay.

And that's just your own personal expenses. Your support team—family, friends, caregivers—may have their own costs: gas, meals, hotel stays, lost wages, and the general wear and tear of helping someone through a major medical event.

At some point, many patients and their families come to a hard realization: "We're going to need help." And just as quickly, a second wave of stress rolls in: *"How do I ask for help without losing my dignity or sound like I am begging?"*

Pride can be a powerful vise. I know that firsthand. There were plenty of times when I made my own life harder because I was too proud to ask for help—even with small things.

It comes down to this —asking for help isn't a failure.

7.2 - The Reality of Transplant Costs

Even with Medicare, private insurance or Medicaid, transplant patients may still face thousands of dollars in out-of-pocket expenses. Insurance may help with the core medical costs, but other essential needs are left uncovered or partially reimbursed.

This isn't a complete list, but here are some of the **most common costs** transplant patients and their families run into:

- Temporary housing near the transplant center (for evaluations, surgery, or recovery)
- Travel expenses for the patient and caregiver (flights, gas, meals, parking, etc.)
- Anti-rejection medications not fully covered by insurance
- Co-pays and deductibles that add up quickly
- Lost wages during recovery—for both patient and caregiver(s)
- Home modifications for safety or mobility (grab bars, ramps, recliners, etc.)
- Additional caregiving costs or in-home help after surgery
- Dental procedures required before approval (yes, even your teeth get judged)
- Ongoing lab work, imaging, and specialist visits

Most patients face these challenges quietly. Some burn through their savings. Some delay care to avoid the financial burden. And far too many try to "tough it out" alone.

7.3 - Reframing the Ask

You know, one of the toughest parts about fundraising isn't setting up a Facebook page or planning a bake sale—it's getting over that uncomfortable feeling of asking for help.

We've all been taught that needing help means you're weak. But really, it takes guts and honesty to say, "Hey, I can't do this by myself."

Try thinking about it differently: fundraising isn't begging—it's inviting people to join your journey.

Most folks don't want to "save" you, but they *will* want to stand beside you, cheer you on, and be part of something that matters. And that's a pretty powerful thing.

You're not selling pity. You're offering purpose. Let people show up for you. And thank them, truly show your appreciation for support.

7.4 - Let Others Host for You

You don't always have to ask directly. In fact, some of the most impactful fundraisers aren't run by the patient at all—they're organized by **friends, family, coworkers, or church members** who care about you and want to help.

When someone else steps up to share your story, it often resonates even more deeply with others.

Here are just a few examples:

- A local BBQ, cookout or community dinner
- A special church offering or donation drive
- A raffle, silent auction, or benefit concert (check laws!!)
- A social media campaign managed by a close friend
- Ask a restaurant if they will donate kitchen space for a 'spaghetti dinner' or 'pancake breakfast' fundraiser.
- If you or a relative is a veteran, you might be able to work with a VFW or American Legion post to host an event.

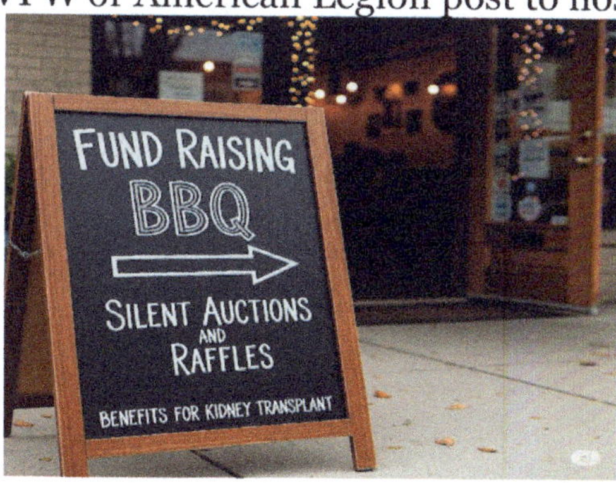
FUND RAISING
BBQ
SILENT AUCTIONS
AND
RAFFLES
BENEFITS FOR KIDNEY TRANSPLANT

7.5 - Offer Something in Return

If asking directly feels awkward or uncomfortable, consider turning your fundraiser into more of an exchange. Giving something back—even something simple or symbolic—can make the process feel more balanced, heartfelt, and even fun. It also gives supporters a tangible way to feel connected to your journey.

Here are a few ideas to spark creativity:

- *Sell t-shirts, wristbands, baked goods, or handmade crafts*. People love a reason to support you—and a keepsake to go with it. Just be sure to factor in all your costs, including shipping and taxes. You don't want to spend $5 to sell it for $5. Be mindful of sales tax and possible business license requirements, though charity fundraisers may have exceptions.

- *Yard sale with a twist.* Host a local yard sale and ask people to donate unwanted item you can sale. I have donated items to neighbors before. Win-Win. I get somethings out of my house, they make money. If it was for a medical fundraiser, I would give even more. (Looking around my house right now, yeah a lot of things I no longer need. Too small to fit clothes come to mind.)

- *Offer personalized digital content* tied to your story or cause—such as behind-the-scenes photos, a short video diary, a mini podcast episode, or a heartfelt article about your experience.

- *Create a "name-a-brick, leaf, or star" option* for larger donations. While symbolic, having their name attached to your journey—a virtual donor wall, a piece of art, or a specific milestone—can be deeply meaningful.

- ***Design a custom digital badge or certificate of appreciation*** for your supporters. It may be a small gesture, but it goes a long way in saying "You mattered to me." They can then share it on social media or simply save it as a reminder that they helped change a life your life.

These gestures don't have to be elaborate. They just need to be real—like you. This approach transforms your ask into a shared experience. It's not a handout—it's a meaningful exchange. And another way to keep your pride intact, while still letting people step in and support you.

One word of caution: Raffles are often considered a form of gambling, so if you're thinking about holding one, don't just double-check—triple-check that it's legal in your city and state.

7.6 - Seek Support from Faith or Community Groups

Churches, temples, mosques, labor unions, and civic clubs often have compassion funds, benevolence ministries, or charitable missions specifically for moments like this.

If you're connected to a group—through faith, work, or your neighborhood—reach out to the leadership. You might be surprised how grateful they might be for the chance to support someone from within their own community.

If you belong to a faith tradition, your request way go beyond finances. You're not just asking for money—you're inviting others into a spiritual partnership. You're asking for prayers, encouragement, and presence during a deeply vulnerable chapter in your life.

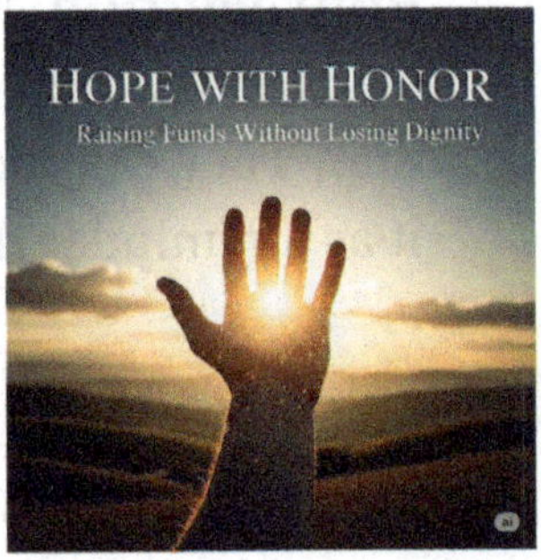

And here's something many people forget: Helping *you* often helps *them* feel useful, connected, and inspired. That's a win-win.

You might even find others who have walked the transplant path themselves who are ready to help you before and afterwards.

Please see Appendix 4 for samples of written requests.

7.7 - Language That Honors Your Story

You may want to include a short message in your fundraiser, email, or flier. Here are a few respectful and warm options:

- "We're walking a hard road. If you'd like to walk it with us, your prayers, shares, and support are deeply appreciated."
- "This transplant is our path back to life, health, and family. We're asking for help from a place of hope."
- "We never expected to be here, but we are here. If you're able to be part of this journey, thank you."

You are loved and supported by many.

Let them be there for you.

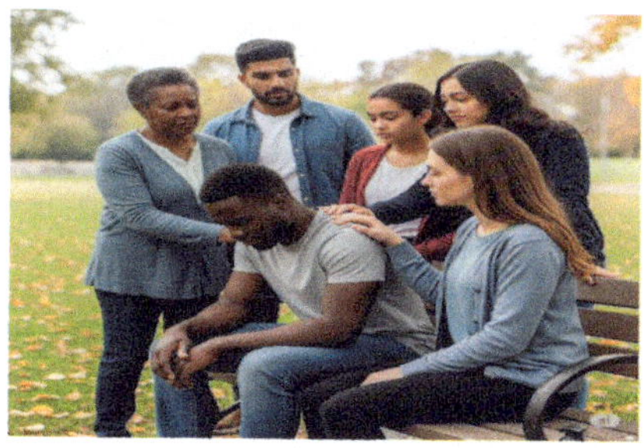

- Commit this to memory:
- You are not just a patient. You are a person.
- You are not a burden. You are a blessing.
- You are not begging. You are building a bridge to life.
- Asking for help isn't the end of dignity—it's the beginning of connections.
- Let people love you. Let them stand with you.
- And let your story be one of strength, not shame.

Chapter 8 -Crowdfunding Tools

This information is provided as a starting point only. I am not endorsing any source, nor do I have personal experience with any of them. Nothing here should be considered legal or financial advice.

Here's a list of a few websites that can help you raise funds :

8.1 - Crowdfunding Platforms (for personal campaigns):

8.1.1 - GoFundMe:

Summary: One of the largest and most well-known crowdfunding platforms, GoFundMe is very popular for medical expenses. It has no platform fees (though payment processing fees apply), offers easy-to-use tools for sharing your story, and provides 24/7 customer support. They also have a donor protection guarantee.

Website: gofundme.com

8.1.2 - FundRazr:

Summary: Designed for social fundraising, FundRazr works well with social media platforms like Facebook. It offers both "keep-it-all" and "all-or-nothing" campaign options. Like GoFundMe, it often has no platform fees but includes payment processing fees.

Website: fundrazr.com

8.1.3 - Fundly:

Summary: Fundly has helped users raise significant amounts of money for various causes. It's user-friendly and accommodates both individuals and nonprofits. Note that some older information suggests they charge a platform fee, so it's essential to verify their current fee structure.

Website: fundly.com

8.1.4 - GoGetFunding:

Summary: This platform features well-designed fundraisers and promotes campaigns on its social media feeds. It accepts major credit cards and processes payments through its in-house system, Stripe, and PayPal, allowing immediate access to donations.

Website: gogetfunding.com

8.1.5 - WhyDonate:

Summary: A platform for medical crowdfunding with a 0% platform fee (only payment processing costs apply). They offer customer support and aim to make it easy to raise money for healthcare emergencies.

Website: whydonate.com

8.2 - Organizations Specializing in Transplant/Medical Fundraising:

8.2.1 - Help Hope Live:

Summary: A national nonprofit organization specifically dedicated to community-based fundraising for medical expenses, including transplants. They offer unique benefits such as keeping your Medicaid/Medicare eligibility, providing personal guidance, and managing funds on your behalf, which can offer peace of mind and tax benefits for donors.

Website: helphopelive.org

8.2.2 - American Kidney Fund (AKF) - KidneyNation:

Summary: The American Kidney Fund is a major organization fighting kidney disease. Through their "KidneyNation" program, you can create a personal fundraising page to raise money to help kidney patients, with a high percentage of funds going directly to programs and patients. They also offer resources and toolkits for effective fundraising.

Website: kidneyfund.org or kidneynation.org

8.2.3 - Children's Organ Transplant Association (COTA):

Summary: Focused on children and young adults (up to age 22), COTA helps families raise funds for transplant-related expenses. With a strong support system, can be a great option if eligible.

Website: cota.org

8.2.4 - National Transplant Assistance Fund (NTAF):

Summary: Similar to Help Hope Live, NTAF is a non-profit that helps patients and families raise funds to cover uninsured medical expenses related to transplantation. They manage funds and ensure compliance with medical and IRS guidelines.

8.3 - Important Considerations for Fundraising:

- Transparency: Be very clear and honest about your situation, what the funds will be used for, and the impact the transplant will have.
- Share Your Story: A compelling personal story with photos can significantly increase engagement and donations.
- Share Widely: Use social media, email, and your personal network to spread the word about your fundraiser.
- Thank Your Donors: Always express gratitude to those who contribute.
- Fees: Be aware of any platform fees and payment processing fees that may reduce the total amount you receive. Some platforms allow donors to cover these fees.
- Tax Implications: For large sums, consult with a financial advisor or tax professional regarding any potential tax implications for received funds. Using a non-profit like Help Hope Live may alleviate some of these concerns for donors as their contributions may be tax-deductible.

Chapter 9 - The Mental Weight Of A Transplant

This isn't just about your body. It's about your head and heart too.

By the time you've made it this far in the process—after labs, interviews, tests, and endless waiting rooms—you might think the biggest challenges are physical. But what no one prepares you for is the mental gymnastics your brain will put you through.

I can tell you firsthand, this isn't a straight path. The emotional terrain is full of potholes and sharp curves. Most you don't even see them coming until you are almost sliding into a ditch.

I would compare the mental journey to driving at night in an extreme snow storm on a narrow winding road where you can see only a few yards in front of the car. You have no idea if there is a curve, a bridge, a stop sign, a stalled car or a tree down across the road.

Why did I say driving at night? Because that is when it will creep into your mind - at night when your room is dark and quiet. When you mind has nothing else to occupy it. Face it head on and don't try to hide from it or let it control you.

9.1 - Before You're Approved: Doubt Creeps In

Once I made the decision to pursue a transplant, I figured it would just be paperwork and patience. What I didn't expect was the internal dialogue that kicked in.

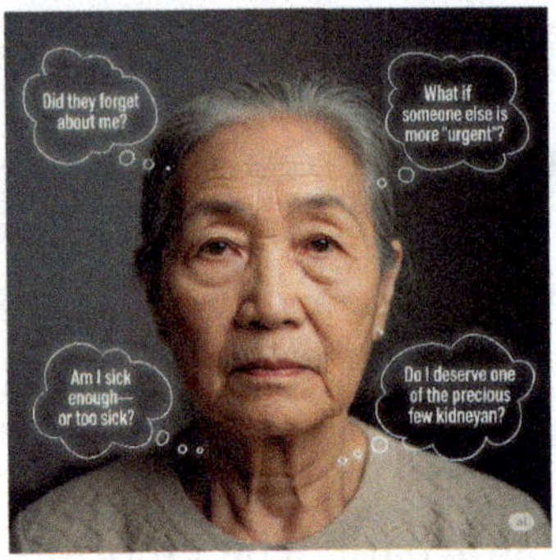

The "what ifs."

- *What if I'm not a good enough candidate?*
- *What if they find something and say no to me being accepted?*
- *Am I wasting everyone's time?*
- *What does it say about me if I'm not chosen?*
- *Do I even deserve one of the few available kidneys?*
- *What if they find another, unknown disease?*

It starts to feel like a judgment—not just on your health, but on your worth. That may sound dramatic to someone on the outside, but it's exactly how it feels when your life depends on someone else's checklist. It's easy to feel exposed and vulnerable, especially when the process isn't moving as fast as your fears are traveling.

You feel like you are trial, the evidence has been presented - and now you are waiting on the verdict from people you don't know to render a decision about your fate. You get no vote. You don't get to be present to argue your case. You can't explain any questions they may have.

You feel hopeful - and - hopeless at the same time.

9.2 - The Waiting Game

Some people get the call in days. Others wait months. I was lucky —my call came fast.

But even in that short window, I had moments where I wondered:

- *Did they forget about me?*
- *What if someone else is more "urgent"?*
- *Am I sick enough—or* ***too*** *sick?*

You're suspended between two lives: the one you're living, and the one you're hoping for. And in that in-between space, doubt moves in, sets up shop in your mind and starts decorating.

9.3 - You Are Not Failing

You will be riding the tilt-a-whirl of emotions—before, during, or after transplant—you are not failing. You're adapting. You're surviving. You're reacting to one of the biggest medical and emotional shake-ups life can throw at you.

Don't compare your journey to anyone else's. Some folks bounce back like a rubber ball. Others feel more like an overcooked noodle—and that's okay.

Some days it'll all make sense. Other days your brain feels like spun cotton candy—light, fluffy, and one step away from disintegrating in the humidity. That's normal too.

Maybe you need time, space, or even a support group to help process it all. There's no prize for pretending to be fine when you're not.

Whatever you're feeling, *feel it*. Then pick yourself up, dust off, and take that next step—wobbly or not. This isn't about being perfect. It's about keeping on, even if you're doing it in mismatched socks and yesterday's pajama pants.

9.4 - The Drive to the Hospital

When the call came, I grabbed my bag, my sister made arrangements for the care of the dog, and we hit the road. I had a two-hour trip with my sister driving. I had nothing to do but sit and think.

And with every mile, my mind threw out every worst-case scenario it could come up with:

- *What if something goes wrong in surgery?*
- *What if the kidney isn't viable after all?*
- *What if this is the end of the road?*
- *What if I wake up in more pain than I imagined? {Note - I did}*
- *What if my body rejects it, even after all this?*
- *Did I forget anything in my legal & medical documents that I need and without they will not proceed.*
- *Did I communicate with everyone I love that I love them?*

Even if you've been calm, focused, and rational so far this could be the moment where fear can crack through the surface. It doesn't make you weak. It makes you human.

I had to remind myself: this is normal. Every person heading into transplant surgery—no matter how brave they look—is carrying questions in the back of their mind.

Chapter 10 - Getting The Call

The phone rings, your heart skips a beat, and suddenly everything becomes very real.

This chapter walks you through what happens when that life-changing call comes in. We'll cover how to prepare a "go bag" with the essentials you'll need. What to expect when you're summoned to the transplant center. The routine check-in procedures and lab work, and finally, being moved into pre-op.

Whether it happens at 3 a.m. or in the middle of a grocery run, you'll be ready to move with calm confidence.

10.1 - Before the call, you should prepare

Recovery from a kidney transplant often only requires a short hospital stay—maybe three to five days—you'll still want to be prepared for comfort, boredom, and maybe a touch of loneliness.

Here's some items for your go-bag:

- **Photo ID and insurance cards**
- **List of emergency contacts**
- **Toothbrush and travel-size toiletries**
- **An up to date list of all current medications**

  Do not take any medications, they will be seized.

- **Legal documents**, including:
    - Health care directives / living will / etc.
    - Power of Attorney (medical and/or general)
    - Organ donor documentation
- **Comfortable, loose-fitting clothing** for the ride home
- **Phone and charger** (an extra long cord is worth AU in a hospital room) High School Chem Test time.
- **Headphones or earbuds** (great for music, calls, or just blocking out noise)
- **Notebook and pen** (jot down questions, reminders, or deep thoughts at 3 a.m.)
- **Lip balm and hand lotion** (hospitals are dry, and so will you be)
- **A book, magazine, or e-reader** for slow hours

And last but not least

- **A stuffed animal, cozy blanket, or comfort item**—yes, even adults get lonely. Bring something soft and familiar. No judgment here.

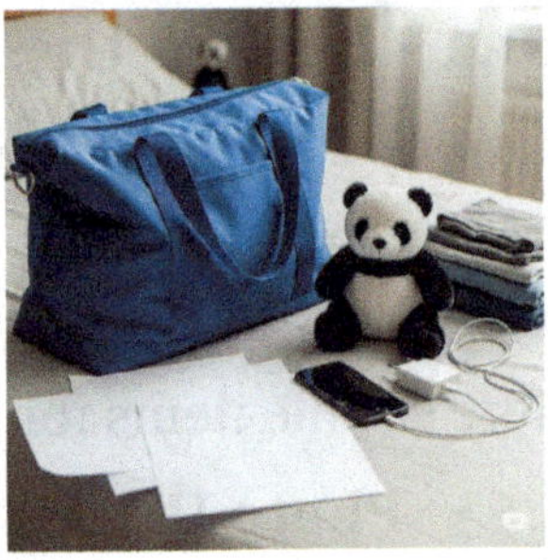

Keep your bag simple and light. A little comfort goes a long way when the world suddenly moves at transplant speed.

Note: The panda has a specific reference but I will only share if you buy me a Thai dinner. hahaha

10.2 - You've been summoned to the transplant center.

This is it—the moment you've been waiting for. Things will start moving quickly now, because the clock is ticking. From the moment a kidney is removed from the donor's body, the countdown begins. Every - Minute - Matters.

The caller will tell you exactly when to arrive and where to go. If after hours, chances are you'll be directed to the ER, as it's typically the only one open. Regardless of where you enter, you'll be checked in and assigned a room for processing. That room could be anywhere in the hospital—whatever is available. It might be in the transplant recovery ward, or it could be a standard hospital room. If in the "Mental Evaluation Wing" you have a whole new set of issues not covered by this handbook.

Once you're settled in, things will start happening—some fast, some slow. You'll go through the usual checks: Blood pressure, Oxygen levels, Pulse, Weight, Blood Glucose levels, etc.

These vitals will be compared to your historical records, looking for anything unusual or concerning. A nurse will also give you a quick covert once or even twice lookie-see. They are checking for open wounds, infections, or anything that might raise a red flag.

This exam is not formal. You might not even realize it's happening—but rest assured, they're observing your physical, emotional, and mental state. Any concerns are quietly relayed to the surgical team.

Next, someone—either a nurse or a lab tech—will draw multiple vials of blood. These will be analyzed and compared to:

- The labs drawn on the day you were first evaluated
- The routine labs from your dialysis center
- Any recent results on file
- Some tests are against the donors blood to check comparability

The goal? Spot any changes that could affect the surgery or anesthesia plan. Your team is looking for signs of infection, clotting issues, or anything that might cause complications.

It's also possible you'll be sent for a quick round of in-hospital dialysis before surgery, depending on test results.

Once medically cleared, you'll be moved to pre-op. Here's where more prep happens:

- IV ports will be placed in multiple spots
- Blood pressure monitors are added
- The octopus of medical sensors are attached

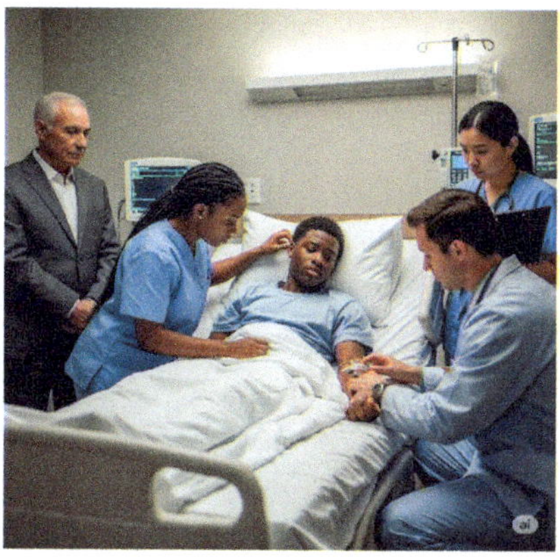

You may receive a visit from multiple members of the surgery team to introduce themselves.

Likely the lead surgical nurse will stop by, at least based on my experiences with major surgeries.

The Anesthesiologist or a team member almost always visits. You can tell how experienced the Anesthesiologist is based on their jokes. The cornier the joke, the longer they been practicing.

My surgeon and a senior surgery resident also stopped by to introduce themselves.

This ensemble of people are not only preparing you medically but they are also working to relieve the stress they know it building up. They know your mind has been bouncing off the walls.

III: Life After Surgery

"Your body has been given a second chance. Now it's your turn to meet it halfway."
— Adapted patient wisdom

This section walks you through the critical days, weeks, and months following your transplant. From medications and medical check-ins to recovery logistics and unexpected complications, you'll get a clear, honest view of what life really looks like after surgery—and how to stay on track for long-term success.

Chapters in this section:

Chapter 1 - Immediately After The Surgery

Your journey isn't over—it's just entering a new phase.

Once your transplant surgery is over, you'll begin the delicate process of recovery.

Your first stop will be Post-Op. This is a critical stop. It is here you will most likely be brought out of the anesthesia induced sleep.

Your time here will be based on many factors including but not limited to:

- Vital Sign Stability – Blood pressure, heart rate, and temperature must be stable and within normal range.
- Pain Management – Pain must be controlled before discharge. (You will still hurt but they want to make sure it is manageable for you once in your recovery room.)
- Psychological Readiness – Anxiety, confusion, or emotional instability may delay discharge to ensure patient safety.
- Bleeding - Signs of any excess bleeding or other surgery related issues.

The Post Op ward nurses will not release you back to your room if there is any fear of complications.

1.2 - Why Dialysis After a Transplant?

Depending on your condition and how things went in the OR, you may be taken directly to your hospital room—or, like me, you might be routed to dialysis first.

This often surprises people. Didn't I just get a kidney to *replace* dialysis? Yes—but here's why a temporary return to the chair may still be necessary:

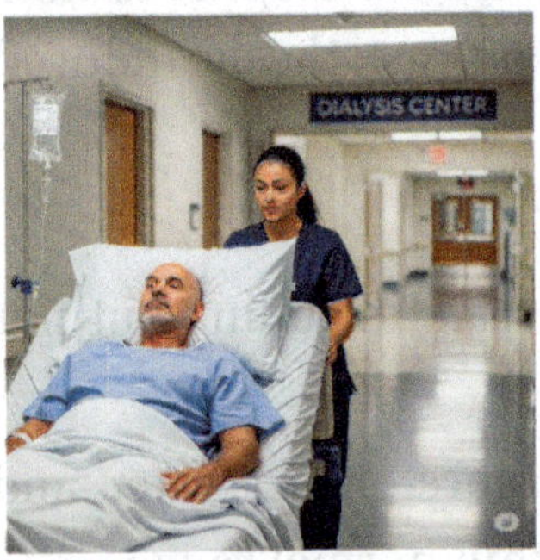

- To remove excess fluids pumped into your body during surgery
- To clear out medications used during the operation
- To reduce elevated potassium levels, which is not uncommon immediately post-op

Additionally, the donor kidney essentially goes to sleep after removal. It needs time—sometimes a day, several days, or even a couple weeks —before it fully wakes up and starts functioning. This is called **delayed graft function**. While it might sound alarming, it's actually pretty normal.

Once that kidney *does* wake up? Watch out. It often goes into overdrive, eager to catch up and flush out the fluids and bi-products buildup in your system. When that happened you will find yourself knowing the exact number of steps between where you are at any minute and the nearest place of accommodation.

1.3 - After Surgery: The Emotional Aftershock

Here's a part almost no one talks about—what happens mentally after the transplant is done.

You wake up sore, foggy, and wondering if you got hit by a truck—or maybe just lost a bar fight you don't remember entering. Distant voices echo like they're from another world (spoiler: it's just the nurses in the hallway). You're hooked to wires, machines are beeping, and your brain is still trying to figure out what day it is.

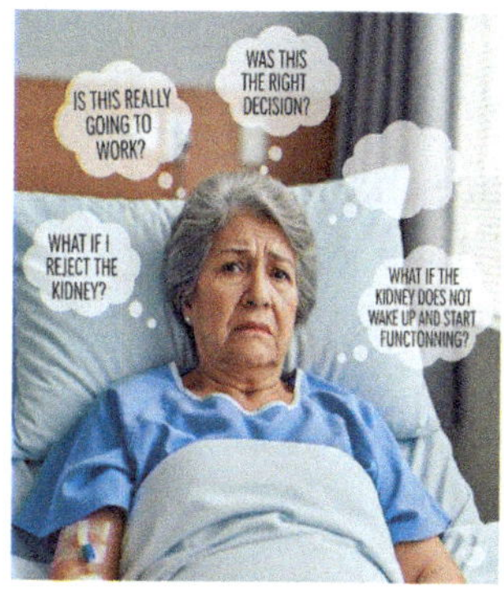

On top of that, your mind starts asking:

- *Is this really going to work?*
- *Was this the right decision?*
- *What if I reject the kidney?*
- *What if the kidney does not 'wake up' and start functioning?*
- *Will there be complications?*
- *Will I be able to afford my medications?*
- *Will my dog still love me?*

I ended up back in the hospital twice with infections. The pain, the setbacks, the slow healing—it was like falling down a flight of stairs and falling back up them for extra effect.

{Those with military experience might have just had flashbacks to Code Reds or Blanket Parties. Not that I would know about those.}

More than once, I grumbled, "This isn't worth it. I was better off on dialysis."

Was that true? Nope. Nada. Zilch.

But it *felt* true at the time. And here's the thing: just because your brain throws a tantrum doesn't mean it's telling the truth. Recovery mess can mess with your body *and* your head. It's a full-contact sport—minus the trophy, but with way more meds.

But it does have cheerleaders. Doctors, specialists, nurses, family and friends. And so you keep playing - if nothing else for them.

1.3.1 - Some Things That Help:

- Journaling — even just a few lines a day
- Talking to other transplant recipients — online or through your center
- Asking your team about a social worker or therapist
- Bringing familiar comforts — music, faith, routines, or yes, even a teddy bear (Panda in my case)
- Reminding yourself — *you've already survived so much*

<table>
<tr>
<td>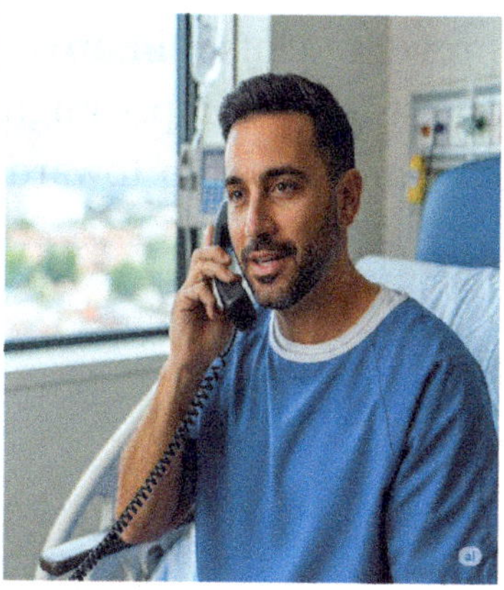</td>
<td>You remember those people who supported you in your journey? The people who helped raise money to help you? One of the most therapeutic things you can do - make a phone call.

It will help you cope with your struggles and let's them know they are appreciated</td>
</tr>
</table>

1.4 - You'll Be Commanded to Walk

Will it hurt? Does a bear....... well, you get the idea.

Nurses will encourage (okay, insist) that you get out of bed and move around, usually within the first 24 hours. Not laps around the hospital—but short, slow, supervised walks with a nurse, a gait belt, and possibly a walker.

But walking is crucial. It helps prevent clots, improves circulation, and speeds up healing. The first few attempts might feel like medieval punishment, but each walk is a step towards going home.

1.5 - The Push to Get You Home

Hospitals try to discharge patients as quickly as safely possible. Once you're stable, with no infection or surgical issues, they'll want you home where you can rest in your own space. Familiar surroundings lift your spirits, and a good mental attitude and altitude will help your body heal faster.

1.6 - After Discharge: The Watchful Weeks

Even after you leave the hospital, you're likely not done with dialysis right away. Until your new kidney starts functioning, you will probably resume your previous dialysis schedule.

You'll also return to the transplant center within a few days for a wound check. The schedule after that depends heavily on your kidney's behavior and your distance from the transplant center.

- If you live close, expect frequent in-clinic visits—possibly every week for a couple months.
- If you live farther away (like I did), the team may set up more often visits by a home health nurse or a wound care center for routine checks. I did make one trip a week for four weeks to the transplant center.

Eventually, home nurse visits will become more common, than in-clinic visits. I had in-home care three times a week for wound checks, vitals, and lab draws. Over time, these visits taper off as your transplant team gains confidence in your recovery.

1.7 - Biopsies: The Follow-Up You Might Not Expect

This is a fairly common procedure done to assess how the transplanted kidney is doing on a microscopic level. They may schedule biopsies:

- **Shortly after transplant**, to establish a baseline
- **Every 6 months to 2 years**, depending on your lab results and medical history

While the word *biopsy* can make people nervous, these are routine and usually outpatient. Just one more piece of the long-term monitoring puzzle.

My kidney wasn't ready to return from vacation when, on March 25, 2020, I went back to the transplant center for an in-clinic wound check and a biopsy. But apparently, the next day, on March 26, the kidney took the biopsy poke as a wake-up call—a time to punch in for work at the local filtration factory.

Coming Up Next: Now that you've made it through surgery and discharge, we'll talk about the transition to life beyond the hospital. Healing, side effects, emotions, labs, new routines—it's a lot, but I will try to present it in manageable nibbles.

Chapter 2 - After Surgery: Housing & Recovery Logistics

The immediate period after transplant surgery is a critical time for healing and recovery. Your living situation plays a significant role in this process. In my personal experience, I was incredibly fortunate to have a sister with ample space and the resources to care for me post-surgery. I discuss this more in Appendix 1.

2.1 - The Transplant Center's Requirements

To be approved for a transplant, the transplant center will require you to have a designated support system for your recovery. This isn't just a suggestion; it's a mandatory part of your application. This short-term support typically lasts at least 30 days, though it could extend for much longer depending on your individual progress.

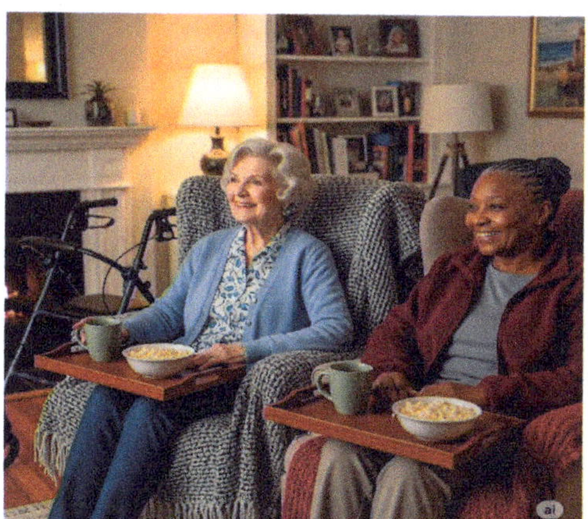

Friends don't let friends recover alone.

During these crucial first weeks, the transplant team does not want you to be alone for extended periods. Their objective is for you to have someone with you most of the time, ideally with no more than four to five hours maximum of solo time – and even less is preferred.

If you have multiple support people, their schedules might be coordinated to ensure continuous coverage. The transplant center will also want to speak with people involved in your in-home support before approving your application. In my case, this was a phone call.

2.2 - Understanding Post-Surgery Limitations

Immediately after surgery, you'll face strict physical restrictions. For example, I was limited to lifting no more than 10 pounds total with both arms combined – roughly the weight of a gallon of milk.

This restriction lasted for several months as my incision healed. Having family support during this time was invaluable; they assisted with everyday tasks like grocery shopping, meal preparation, laundry, and other household chores that become challenging when you can't lift or strain.

Meals in bed were not provided. I was sternly informed I needed to walk and walking to the table was important.

2.3 - Essential Home Care Needs

Beyond physical assistance, your in-home support person plays a vital role in monitoring your recovery. Two of the most important aspects of post-transplant care at home are:

- Watching for possible bleeding.
- Ensuring you're eating and drinking properly
- Verifying you are consistently taking all required medications.
- Enforcing a limited exercise program is also important – even if just walking in the house.

At various points in the recovery and wound healing process, you might also need assistance with wound care, which could be managed at home by your support person or require visits to a clinic.

Having a robust and reliable support system in place is not just a convenience; it's a fundamental component of a successful and safe recovery journey.

Chapter 3 - The Meds You'll Take For Life

Please note: As previously stated in Disclaimers, my cocktail combination likely will differ from you patients.

I am going to break this discussion in to three main groups with sub-groups as needed.

(1) Transplant specific medications

(2) Regular prescriptions from you personal doctors.

(3) OTC, Over-The-Counter

3.1 - Staying On Top Your Medications Schedule

It might feel overwhelming—25 medications, a dozen reminders, and a schedule that never seems to quit. But this isn't just about pills and charts.

Every dose, every check-in, every "yes" to your care plan is an investment in your future. It's how you give yourself the best shot at being there—really *being there*—for the people who matter most.

Taking care of yourself is your full-time job now, and sure, it's a big one. But it's also an act of love—love for yourself, and love for those who are counting on you to stick around, healthy and strong

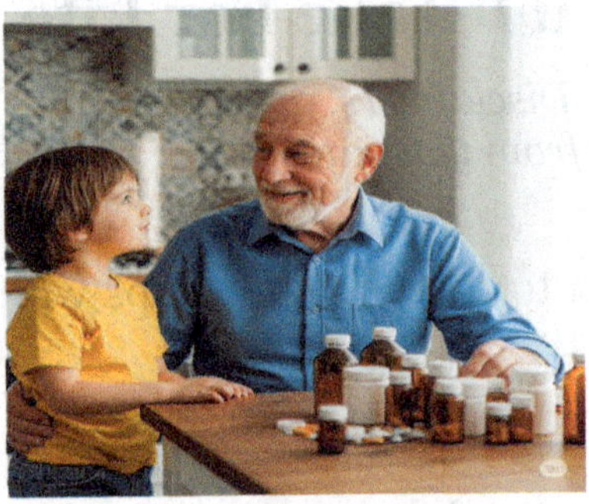

Every dose you take is a small promise kept to those who are cheering you on—like a grandchild who still needs your stories, your hugs, and just your presence.

Before you panic over 25 medications, 3 or 4 is the average transplant-specific medications. Counting OTC vitamins - I take 8 daily different items, only 3 are anti-rejection.

I wanted to get your attention with that many medications to stress the importance of being mindful of the obligation.

3.2 - Navigating Medications: Your Lifelong Partnership

The human body possesses an astonishing self-healing and protective capability. It instinctively mends wounds, from a tiny scratch to even fending off invading organisms like cold viruses. You are, in essence, born with a sophisticated natural defense system designed to rid your body of anything "not original equipment".

But, if the body receives something truly beneficial, like a kidney, lung, heart, personality - that same powerful immune system sees it as a "foreign invader". This a natural instinct to fight it.

Thanks to decades of medical research, advanced anti-rejection drugs (also known as immunosuppressants) have greatly reduced complications and deaths, making organ transplants a life-saving reality for millions. Every year brings stronger treatments and smarter drugs. Side effects drop. Risks shrink. Compatibility improves.

The road ahead? Brighter than ever.

3.2.1 - Your Initial Medication Regimen

Right after your transplant, you'll take a mix of medications—some short-term, others for life. Early on, several are vital to help your body accept the new organ as it heals.

I started on transplant and surgery related medications:

- Three anti-rejection medications
- One anti-viral medication (phased out in months)
- One anti-bacterial medication (phased out in months)
- Vitamin D
- **A laxative:** This was important because some transplant medications, as well as powerful pain and anesthesia medications used during surgery, can cause constipation.

3.2.2 - The Evolving Anti-Rejection Medication Schedule

Managing anti-rejection medications is a dynamic process, often requiring careful adjustments over time:

- **Tapering:** One of my three anti-rejection medications had a built-in "step-down" schedule over several months. My doctors reduced it ahead of the typical schedule, even cutting it to half the average normal dosage.
- **Sudden changes:** Another remained consistent until a serious, transplant-related infection led to my second hospitalization. That particular prescription was temporarily stopped while I was on other medications for the infection. It was restarted once the infection was gone.
- **Fine-tuning:** The third anti-rejection compound was adjusted frequently in the beginning. As often as every couple of weeks before settling down at about 6 months.

It continues to be adjusted a few times a year. That's why it's essential to stay on top of your standing lab orders. Doctors aim to keep certain readings within target ranges, adjusting dosages as needed. It might feel annoying, but tweaking meds every few months is still better than sitting in a dialysis chair every few days.

3.2.3 - Managing Your Medication Schedule

Following your transplant, you should receive a clear, personalized sheet listing all your medications and a daily schedule (e.g., "First in the morning," "one hour later," "mid-day," "evening," "bedtime"). For me, it simplified to three main time slots: early morning, one hour later, and then exactly 12 hours after that second morning dose, ensuring consistent 12-hour spacing between certain medications. It's highly advisable to fill out this sheet in **pencil**, allowing for easy updates as your dosages inevitably change.

3.2.4 - Specialty Pharmacies and Delivery Logistics

Most transplant medications are obtained through specialty pharmacies linked to or contracted by your transplant center. These are usually mail-order, with 30-day supplies due to high costs and insurance limits. Because of their value and potency, they may require secure, direct delivery to you rather than a third party

This strict delivery protocol is also an important consideration when discussing travel restrictions. I schedule my trips around my refill schedule.

3.3 - Regular Prescriptions: Beyond Immunosuppression

Along with transplant-specific drugs, you may continue or start other prescriptions for overall health. For example, I kept my statin and low-dose aspirin after surgery, and later added blood pressure medication—prescribed by the transplant team but now managed by my primary care doctor.

These regular medications are usually widely available and often supplied in 90-day amounts. Both my PCP and transplant center can order them through my local pharmacy.

You can also use mail-order services like Amazon PillPack or Express Scripts instead of a local pharmacy. These are especially helpful for managing multiple meds and often offer cheaper 90-day supplies compared to 30-day local fills.

3.4 - Over-the-Counter (OTC) Medications: Proceed with Caution

When it comes to over-the-counter (OTC) medications and supplements, never add or stop anything without first consulting your transplant team. I also make sure to clear anything significant with my PCP.

This strict rule is vital because some OTC treatments can interfere with anti-rejection drugs, reducing their effectiveness or causing harmful side effects.

For kidney transplant recipients, common pain relievers like Advil (ibuprofen) and other NSAIDs can harm the kidneys. This limits safe pain relief options mainly to Tylenol (acetaminophen) and its generics. Even then, caution is essential—never exceed recommended doses or use it long-term, as it can affect the liver.

From personal experience, when my Optometrist suggested a vitamin routine like AREDS (e.g., Bausch & Lomb PreserVision), my first step was to email both my PCP and transplant team. Without their approval, I wouldn't start. Thankfully, they gave the green light.

Summary: Your Central Clearing Point

The key rule for all medications and supplements—prescribed or OTC—is to never make changes without consulting your transplant center first. Also, check with any other primary care specialists you see.

Even if another doctor prescribes a medication, your transplant team should remain your central "clearing point" for all medical decisions. This careful coordination is essential to protect your new organ and your overall health.

Chapter 4 - Testing, Labs, and Constant Check-Ins

Life after transplant surgery introduces a new set of routines crucial for monitoring your health and the new organ's function. This involves two distinct, yet ultimately intertwined, activities: diligent **daily record-keeping** at home and **regularly scheduled medical lab tests**.

While one is a daily patient responsibility and the other involves a medical facility, both become an integral part of your life as a transplant recipient.

4.1 - Daily Record-Keeping: Your At-Home Command Center

Upon discharge, your medical team will provide specific instructions for closely monitoring key vital statistics.

The chart I was provided initially requested daily readings for:

- Weight: Once a day
- Temperature: Twice a day
- Blood Pressure (B/P): Three times a day
- Heart Rate/Pulse: Three times a day
- Glucose: Four times a day (if diabetic)

By carefully recording these vitals each day, potential issues can be spotted early—often before they escalate into serious problems. Just as diabetics are accustomed to frequent glucose checks, transplant patients adapt to a similar vigilance.

As a non-diabetic, I customized my chart to remove the glucose readings. Embracing my "computer geekness", I created a spreadsheet with a page for each month, adding columns for O2 saturation and notes. Being computerized it was extremely more readable than my penmanship plus easy to email my care team.

It only takes a few minutes a day and offers significant peace of mind. Beyond transplantation, this daily tracking is also an excellent proactive measure for anyone concerned about the flu, COVID, West Nile Virus, or other viral events—a simple way to spot potential problems early.

4.2 - Regularly Scheduled Labs: Your Medical Checkpoints

Regular laboratory testing generally falls into two main groups, though the specific tests and their frequency will vary between patients and can change based on individual needs or random medical assessments.

My key regular tests include Tacrolimus (Tacro) levels, a Hematology & Coagulation Panel (CBC with Diff), and a Renal Panel. Other tests in the past have included BK Virus, Glucose Stress, and Epstein-Barr. Before you cancel your Bacon King Whopper - BK is not for Burger King.

In practice, my role is simple: I go to the lab, a skilled technician draws my blood, and the samples are sent for testing. What exactly is tested isn't my immediate concern—my job is to keep my appointments. The lab ensures accurate processing, and the doctors interpret the results.

I make it a point to have my lab orders sent directly to me and carry a physical copy. While most patients rely on the clinic to receive them, having my own copy has saved me when the clinic's computers aren't cooperating.

A crucial note: some lab tests cannot be drawn if you've taken certain medications before the test. You will need to pay very careful attention to specific instructions from your medical team.

Additionally, a few labs may require fasting prior to the test. Be aware that both situations—withholding a medication dose or fasting—may apply to different tests.

My lab schedule started pretty intense—twice a week for the first month. As things stabilized, it eased to weekly, then every two weeks, and finally monthly. For some, labs might stretch out to every two or three months, but that really depends on each person's situation. If something unusual shows up, a quick follow-up test might be needed right away.

Lab schedules are about as predictable as the weather! For example, I stayed on monthly labs longer due to complications, and after a serious infection, I went back to weekly labs for a while. Thankfully, during that time, a home healthcare nurse drew my blood, so I didn't have to travel to the hospital.

My best advice regarding changes in blood lab testing schedules? Don't stress over it; just roll with it. Flexibility is key in managing post-transplant care.

Chapter 5 - The Not-So-Fun Stuff That Might Happen

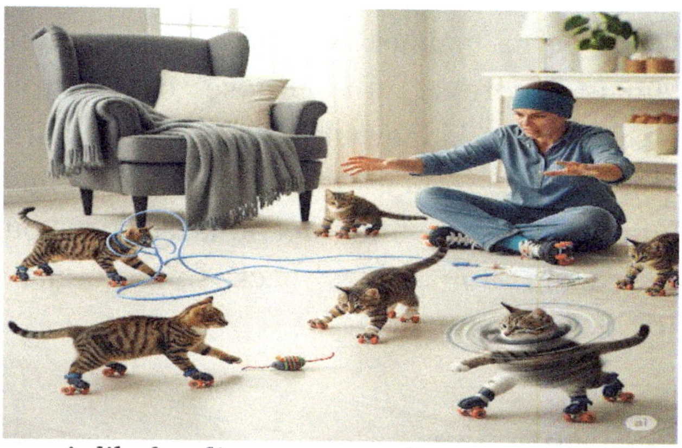

"Recovery is like herding cats on roller skates. Looks fun on paper."

So you survived transplant surgery. High five! (Okay, gentle elbow bump – you're still healing.) Now comes the next stage of the journey: recovery. Some people heal like they've got superhero DNA. Others? Let's just say recovery can feel like a game of "Whack-a-Mole" and you are the table – and life brought a bigger hammer.

You can expect an average of 6–8 months for most of the wound to heal. Could be sooner. Could be longer.

Because of a re-infection towards the end, my recovery was closer to 14 months. I say this not to scare you but assure you, I was a major exception and if you are one also, just understand, it is nothing personal - just a part of life. U of M took care of me.

5.1 - The Not-So-Fun Stuff That Might Happen

5.1.1 - Infections.

You'll feel like a germ magnet – and you kinda are. Your immune system is suppressed on purpose to keep your body from attacking your new kidney like it's a college dorm party crasher. So even a sneeze from a toddler could turn into a 3-day vacation at Hotel Hospital. Wound infections, airborne bugs, and anything your cousin Bob brings back from a gas station bathroom – it's all fair game.

5.1.2 - Bladder Confusion.

Picture your bladder as a sleepy security guard who suddenly got a promotion to night manager. It's undertrained and overworked. It hasn't done anything useful in a while, and now it's asked to perform on command. Result? Frequent small bathroom trips.

5.1.3 - Stuck Urethra

Sometimes the urethra just doesn't get the memo. In those cases, the catheter might make a guest appearance. No one likes it – not even the nurses. But if it helps, think of it as temporary plumbing until the system figures itself out.

5.2 - Recovery Routette

Even with all the right meds, clean living, and monk-level hygiene, some folks just hit snags. But here's the thing: the success rate for kidney transplants in the U.S. is remarkably high. We're talking well over 90% one-year survival for most patients. Depending on donor type (living donor vs deceased) and the transplant centers quality, survival rates can be 97-99%. That's not just good — that's strong reason to have the faith and determination to complete your transplant efforts.

Sure, it might take some adjustments. Some setbacks might surprise you. And some days you'll just feel "off" — like your body is buffering. But this isn't a sprint. It's a slow jog through a medical obstacle course with hydration stations and lab work checkpoints.

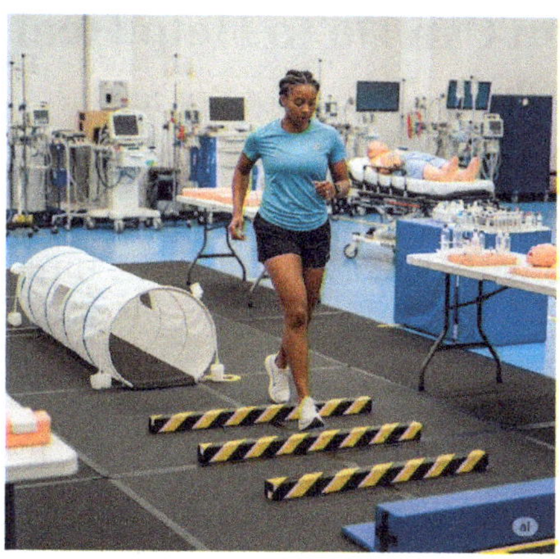

5.3 - Psychological and Emotional Well-being:

Stress, anxiety, and depression can affect a person's ability to stick to their medical regimen and lifestyle changes, indirectly slowing or complicating recovery. When mental health takes a hit, it's harder to remember medications, follow dietary rules, attend appointments, or even care about long-term outcomes.

Emotional strain can impact sleep, appetite, energy levels, and immune response—all critical to post-transplant healing. This is why mental health care isn't a luxury—it's part of your treatment. Whether it's therapy, peer support, spiritual guidance, or medication, finding the right support system can protect both your transplant and your quality of life.

5.4 - Things You Can Do to Help Heal

(Besides Praying and Not Screwing It Up)

The surgery's done. You've got a shiny new organ, a head full of questions, and a body that feels like it went three rounds with a linebacker.

Congrats—you've made it to the part where healing becomes your full-time job. The doctors probably handed you a binder thicker than a phone book—or for those too young to remember phone books, imagine printing out your cellphone's license agreement. Yeah, that thick.

But even with all that info, no one really tells you what it *feels* like to be home with your new plumbing. Post-transplant recovery isn't just about lying around watching daytime TV (though that's part of it). It's about *active healing*—doing your part to protect this incredible gift. Prayers help, but here are a few real-world steps you can take to keep things on track.

5.4.1 - Medication Adherence: This isn't the time to get creative. You're not baking banana bread and wondering if nutmeg would add a twist. Take your meds. Exactly as prescribed. Every. Single. Time.

5.4.2 - Diet: Yes, we all want comfort food. But guess what's not comforting? Kidney rejection.

Stick to the low-sodium, low-fat life — not because it's fun, but because it works. Avoid grapefruit and pomegranate. They sound innocent, but they're drug-sabotaging little devils.

And let's not pretend gas station sushi is ever a good idea. Food safety matters now more than ever — your immune system is working part-time, and raw chicken isn't a joke anymore.

5.4.3 - Physical Activity: We're talking light walking, not CrossFit. No, you don't "got this bro." Save the heroic lifting for the next Marvel movie. Your job is to move gently, stretch a little, and not pop a stitch. Walking is great. If you're sweaty and breathless, you went too far. Back it up, champ.

5.4.4 - Fluid and Hydration: Hydrate like your kidney depends on it — because it does. Water is medicine. Initially you may get tired of peeing every 40 minutes, but hey, that's actually a win in the transplant world. Eventually your bladder will expand, reducing your need to visit the facilities as often.

5.4.5 - Existing Health Conditions: Don't ignore the stuff that got you here in the first place. High blood pressure and diabetes are not background characters — they could have been villains in this sequel. Keep them in check or they'll rewrite the whole story.

5.5 - Set Up A Schedule Checklist For Each Daily Task

Following a strict schedule goes against my norm. Maybe it's just me getting old and cantankerous—although, to be fair, some folks *erroneously* claim I was cantankerous long before I had the "old" part going for me. Still, I like having no fixed schedule.

But 11 years on dialysis, 3 times a week was a schedule I hated a lot more I have now. Like it or not, it *is* important to stick to a schedule. That means staying on top of your medications, getting decent food and nourishment, drinking enough water, and yes... the Evil "E" word: Exercise. You don't have to like it. You just have to do it.

(Grumbling optional.)

Chapter 6 - Post-Op Wound Treatments You Might Use

Welcome to the fine art of belly feng shui: gauze here, tape there, antiseptic cream in area three of the abdominal arts district, sterile vibes only. No duct tape, super glue or all weather caulk permitted.

While this guide focuses on kidney transplants, the topic of wound care crosses into many types of major surgeries and wounds. From a kidney transplant, vascular access revision, or other surgical procedures, understanding how to care for open or partially healed wounds is critical.

This chapter offers an abbreviated overview of post-surgical wound treatment methods you may encounter. These are not universal nor are they absolutely inclusive. Treatments used for your wound(s) can vary greatly. Always follow the guidance of your surgeon or wound care team.

Wound healing is a complex, multi-stage process that's highly individualized. No one-size-fits-all solution exists. Wound care is it's own medical specialty. Trust your provider is tailoring the treatment to your body's specific needs at each phase, and don't hesitate to ask questions along the way.

I discussed in Appendix A, what my team used.

I apologize in advance about some of these illustrations. I felt a picture explained better than words.

6.1 - Wound Vac Systems (Negative Pressure Wound Therapy)

A wound vac system is a portable, battery-powered device designed to promote wound healing through negative pressure. The system includes a specialized foam or other porous packing material inserted into the wound, which is then sealed with an airtight bandage. The base unit, typically carried by the patient, creates suction by removing air from the wound site. It also draws out wound discharge into container for safe disposal.

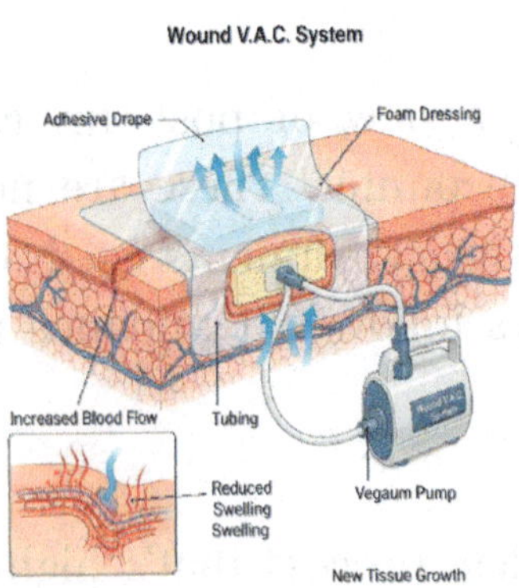

The negative pressure does more than just keep the wound clean. It stimulates increased blood flow to the wound area. The blood delivers oxygen and nutrients essential for cellular regeneration. This enhanced circulation accelerates healing and helps the edges of the wound draw together, encouraging the tissue to close naturally.

Wound vac dressings are typically changed 2 or 3 times a week—either in the transplant center, at a wound care clinic, or by a certified home healthcare provider. They should not be changed by the patient or by uncertified individuals. The treatment continues until the wound has healed sufficiently and becomes too small to accommodate the foam packing.

6.2 - PICO System (Mini Wound Vac Therapy)

The PICO System—while technically a brand name—is often used as a shorthand to describe using any of the smaller, more compact versions of a wound vac. Like people say Scotch Tape but are referring to any clear tape.

This miniaturized device operates on the same general principle as a full-sized wound vac: it applies negative pressure to the wound site to promote faster healing. However, it comes in a much smaller package—roughly the size of a pack of cigarettes—and is fully battery operated.

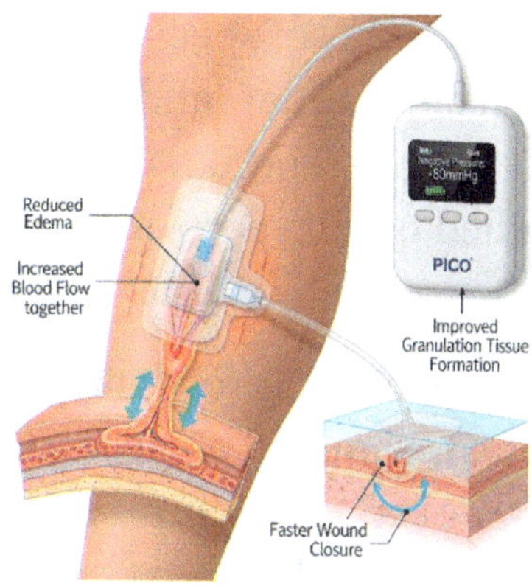

Unlike larger wound vac units, the mini-systems are designed to last up to a week with intervention. It's commonly applied and removed by a wound care specialist, although a nurse may also handle removal if needed. The device operates the same as the wound vac, just on a smaller-scale.

A mini-system is used during the later stages when the wound no longer requires as much suction effort but still benefits from the continued application of negative pressure.

6.3 - Wound Healing Assistance Pads

Wound healing assistance pads come in many variations and formulations. These are typically used in the final stages of wound care, when the wound is technically still open but has become very small and shallow.

Some of these specialized pads may only be available by a physician's order and administered under the guidance of a wound care specialist. Occasionally some treatments can be handled by a layperson once shown the proper steps.

The application process is relatively straightforward. A portion of the pad, trimmed as necessary, is placed directly into or over the wound bed. It's covered with a secondary dressing–such as gauze or an absorbent pad to hold it in place and absorb any minor discharge. These pads often contain antimicrobial agents like silver (as in "AG" products), foam layers to manage moisture, or gel to promote healing in low-exudate wounds.

They serve as a bridge between active wound therapy and complete closure, helping ensure the last stages of healing occur safely and without infection.

Before you reach for your copy of Merck Manual of Diagnosis and Therapy, a low-exudate wound is one that doesn't leak much fluid. They usually stay dry and need gentle care to help them heal.

6.4 - Wet-to-Dry Dressings

A *wet-to-dry* dressing is a traditional wound care method used to help clean and promote healing in moderate to heavily draining wounds. The process saline moistened sterile gauze placed directly in the wound. It is covered it with a dry gauze or outer dressing to keep it in place. Holding this together is medical tape. Having a reaction to some different types of tape - I used silk surgical tape. This tape is very clingy - and will remove hair on par with a waxing, or so I have been told.

The purpose of the moist gauze is twofold: it keeps the wound environment damp—which can aid in healing—and it helps draw out wound discharge or debris as the gauze dries. When the dressing is removed, it can also take some of that drainage and dead tissue with it. The gauze acts as form of debridement (a medical procedure meaning to remove dead, damaged, or infected tissue from a wound).

Wet-to-dry dressings are relatively simple and can be applied by a healthcare professional or, once trained, by the patient or a caregiver. Frequency of dressing changes varies depending on the wound's condition and may range from multiple times per day to just a few times per week.

Though not as common in modern advanced wound care (due to more specialized products), wet-to-dry remains a reliable and accessible option—especially in home care or transitional wound management settings.

6.5 - Open but Covered

At certain points in the healing process—or even between other types of treatments—a wound care specialist may recommend keeping a wound *open but covered*. In this case, the wound is no longer packed with dressings or wound products but is still protected with a sterile outer covering, like a simple gauze pad or breathable dressing.

The goal here is to allow the wound to "breathe" without exposing it to dirt, friction, or outside contaminants. This method is often used when the deeper tissue layers have started to heal and new skin (epithelium) has begun to form over the wound bed. The wound may still be fragile and this type of coverage helps keep it clean and moist enough to continue healing without interference.

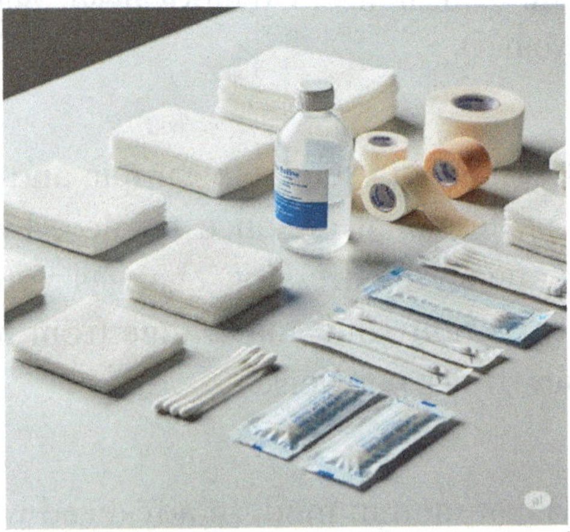

I still have a small supply of wound care at my house

6.6 - Hydrocolloid Dressings

- These gel-like dressings interact with the moisture in the wound to create a healing environment.
- They're used for superficial wounds or surgical sites with minimal drainage.
- Often left in place for 3–5 days and removed by a nurse or patient under supervision.

6.7 - Silicone Gel Sheets

- Used once a wound is closed to reduce scarring or treat hypertrophic scars.
- They provide a soft covering that helps flatten raised scars and maintain skin moisture.
- Can be reused for several weeks; typically recommended by plastic surgeons or transplant teams concerned about long-term cosmetic outcomes.

6.8 - Steri-Strips or Surgical Tape

- Thin adhesive strips used to reinforce healing incisions once stitches are removed.
- They help keep the skin edges together and reduce stress on the healing tissue.
- They usually fall off on their own but can be gently removed after a week if instructed.

6.9 - Antibiotic Ointments or Medicated Creams

- Sometimes used in very small amounts to prevent localized infections.
- Often phased out once the wound begins to close to avoid slowing healing .
- Usually used only in the early days of healing.
- Overuse can delay healing or irritate skin.

Final Thoughts

Wound care may not be the most glamorous part of recovery, but it plays a huge role in how smoothly things go—and how quickly you get back to life. Each of these treatments has its own purpose and place, and it's not uncommon to use more than one type throughout the healing process.

The best part? You're not expected to figure this out on your own. You'll have a care team watching closely, guiding your next steps, and adjusting your treatment as your body moves forward. Ask questions, stay involved, and trust that even slow healing is still healing.

Chapter 7 - Meet Your New BFFs

You thought your best friend was the person who held your hair back during that one regrettable night in 2006? Cute, but wrong. Post-transplant, your *real* ride-or-die buds are wearing scrubs, carrying clipboards, have stethoscopes and asking you awkward questions about your bathroom habits.

These dedicated folks are your health team, your guides, and your biggest cheerleaders on this recovery journey. You might not see them at your birthday party, but they'll definitely be there when it counts.

Thanks to the greatest thing since the greatest thing since sliced bread - video visits - many doctor appointments are possible remotely.

This separately begs the question, what was the greatest thing before sliced bread became the greatest thing?

7.1 - Your Primary Care Physician

Chances are, you already have a relationship with your primary care physician (PCP). After your transplant, that relationship may become a bit more involved — and that's a good thing.

Your PCP also becomes the point person for any new or unrelated medical issues that come up, and it's crucial that your transplant team stays in the loop about those also.

While your transplant team will handle most of the early medications and follow-ups, some of those prescriptions may eventually be transferred to your PCP for monitoring and refills.

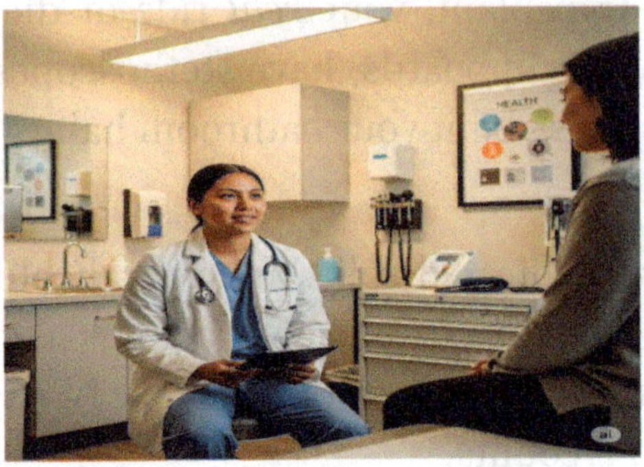

Thanks to today's interconnected medical systems, there's a good chance your transplant center is part of a larger hospital network. If your PCP is also in a healthcare system with electronic medical records, those networks may "talk" to each other. This can streamline your care by keeping all your providers aware of what medications you're on or what therapies you're undergoing.

That said, not all systems share everything, and not all details are visible across platforms. So, even with fancy tech in place, a little human follow-up never hurts. You might still need to confirm details with your transplant coordinator or bring copies of records with you.

7.2 - Your Dentist

Oral health has always mattered – but after a transplant, it becomes even more important. Your mouth isn't just for smiling and talking; it's also a primary gateway into your body. Bacteria that build up in your gums or teeth can travel into the blood system. This may cause serious complications, especially when your immune system is dialed down by medications.

Regular dental exams and professional cleanings aren't just for fresh breath and white teeth anymore. They're a vital part of your overall health. Catching a cavity early or treating gum inflammation before it spreads can make a real difference in preventing bigger issues down the line.

Let your dentist know you're a transplant recipient and what medications you're on so they can take that into account during treatment. Some transplant centers even recommend or even require getting a dental clearance as part of your pre-transplant evaluation.

If any oral surgeries or other serious dental work is expected, the transplant care team should be coordinated with as there might be unpleasant medications interactions.

7.3 - Your Transplant Nephrologist

Think of your transplant nephrologist as the quarterback of your kidney care team — especially in the months after surgery. This is the doctor who specializes in how your new kidney is doing, how well it's functioning, and what tweaks might be needed to keep it working smoothly for as long as possible.

Unlike your surgery team (who you may only see a few times post-op), your transplant nephrologist is in it for the long haul. They'll monitor lab results, track your numerous test result levels, adjust your meds, and watch for signs of rejection or infection. They're also the ones who help you strike that delicate balance between preventing rejection and keeping your immune system strong enough to handle everyday life.

Expect to see your transplant doctor regularly — more frequently right after surgery, then gradually tapering off to a manageable rhythm if everything goes well. They'll often be your go-to for interpreting labs, making medication changes, and coordinating with your primary care physician or other specialists when something unexpected shows up.

Your relationship with your transplant center may be one of the most important and longest-lasting connections in your post-transplant life. It's okay to ask questions, push for explanations, and work together to understand how your kidney is doing — after all, you're a team now.

7.4 - Your Regular Nephrologist

Before your transplant, your kidney doc and their crew were your go-to team while on dialysis. After the big surgery, that doesn't change—it just shifts gears.

The first year, the transplant center runs point. They keep a close eye on things providing updates to your regular nephrologist. Later, your hometown kidney doc gets back in the saddle. Think of it like co-pilots: the transplant team handles the special stuff, and your regular doc makes sure everything else runs smooth. Both are important to keep the kidney chugging along.

The good news is the two doctors will work together to manage your care. The bad news, unlike your parents, you can't get away with stuff by saying the other one said it was okay.

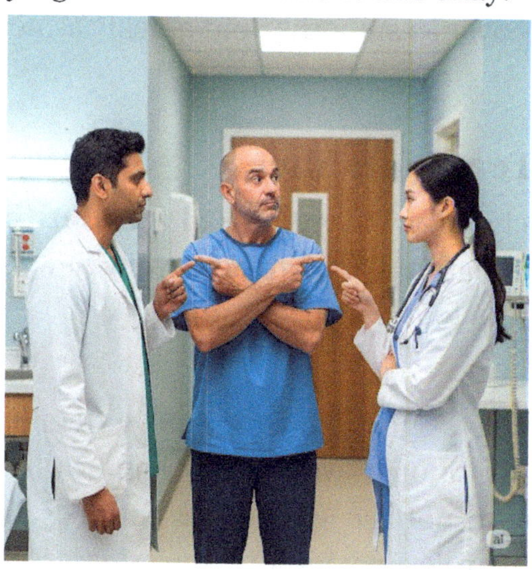

7.5 - Wound Care Specialist

As part of your post-surgery recovery, you may be referred to a wound care specialist. Healing after transplant surgery doesn't always follow a neat, straight line.Having experts focused solely on wound healing can make a big difference in both your comfort and your recovery time.

Wound care specialists are up to date on the latest techniques and therapies for helping surgical sites heal properly. In my case, my wound care team included a Physician Assistant and a couple attentive nurses who worked with me regularly for a couple months.

If you do end up needing wound care, know that you're in good hands. These teams are skilled, encouraging, and focused on helping you recover as smoothly and quickly as possible.

7.6 - Misc Team Members

You'll also likely talk with a **transplant dietitian**, who'll help you adjust your eating habits to keep your new kidney happy — think of them as a food coach.

There will also be a **transplant social worker.** They can help support your emotional well-being, help with resources, and make sure you're not navigating this journey alone. Both play small but mighty roles in your long-term success.

7.7 - Home health care nurses

I saved the best for last — and with good reason.

It's very likely you'll be assigned a home health care provider transplant before your initial discharge. These are normally Registered Nurses (RNs) or Licensed Practical Nurses (LPNs). They may visit as often as three times a week, weekly, or just every other week.

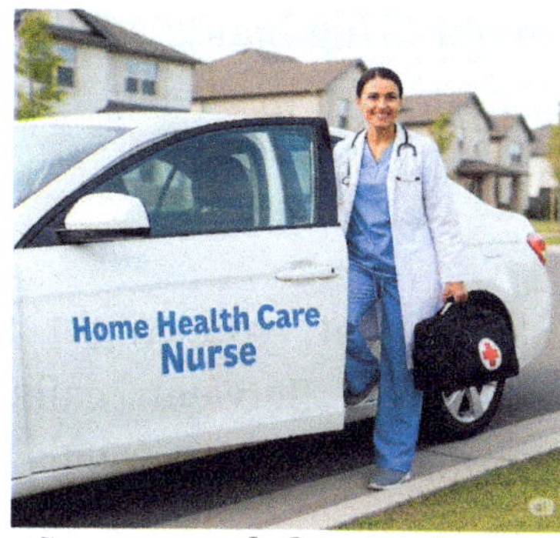

Some angels have wings some have tires

That frequency, paired with the very personal nature of the care they provide, builds a strong and trusting bond. They're there not just to take vitals, change dressings, or help with medications – they become your front line of care. You'll quickly come to appreciate their skill, their presence, and the comfort of knowing someone truly has your back conveniently in your own home. Mine explained things about wound care and even lab tests when I was confused.

And if you want to make a friend for life, at the end of your wound care – gift them any donate any extra supplies. They often have a small stock in their car for patients that need things the patient does not have. That stock saved me a couple times!!

Wrapping Up the Care Team

Just when you think the parade's over – surprise! A Physical or Occupational Therapist might show up to help you get your strength and mobility back. They're the "back-on-your-feet" crew – might bring bands, walkers, or even suggest moving the couch so you don't trip over it. Their visits may be short, but their help sticks with you.

At this point, you might feel like your living room needs a receptionist. Between calls from the transplant center, visits from nurses and therapists, it's like hosting a small-town clinic at home.

Yep, it's a lot. But every one of 'em is part of the same mission: getting you stable, stronger, and back to living with your new kidney. And hey – with all these folks stopping by, you'll never forget how to give addresses to your house.

IV: Adjusting to a New Norm

"Sometimes the hardest part isn't surviving the storm—it's learning to live after it."
— J.M. Storm

This section focuses on life beyond the hospital walls—where healing meets everyday living. You'll learn how to care for your new kidney through smart eating, clean habits, safe travel, and balanced socializing. Whether you're easing back into public spaces or finding support online, this is about building a life that protects your health without putting your joy on pause.

Chapters in this section:

1. Eating for Your New Kidney
2. Sanitation Without Paranoia
3. Getting Out There After Transplant
4. Helping Others While Helping Yourself
5. Support Groups Online

Chapter 1 - Eating for Your New Kidney

Your new kidney is working hard to help you heal—and what you put on your plate makes a big difference. In the weeks and months after surgery, your body needs more protein than usual to repair the surgical site, support wound healing, and rebuild muscle.

Lean meats, poultry, fish, eggs, and dairy can all be part of your recovery plan, <u>if</u> they fit in your personal desires and your body can handle them. i.e. Lactose Intolerant or a Vegan.

If you remember when first facing dialysis, you had to learn to read ingredient labels extremely careful. After time, you stopped reading most labels because you already knew what they said - what ingredients where contained.

Now is the time to refresh your reading skills. It may not be as important in many ways, in other ways, it might be more. Broken record time - your dietitian is your best source for foods that are bad and could cause problems with your medications

The goal is simple: give your kidney the best environment to thrive while you regain strength and confidence in your daily life.

1.1 - Fueling Your New Life

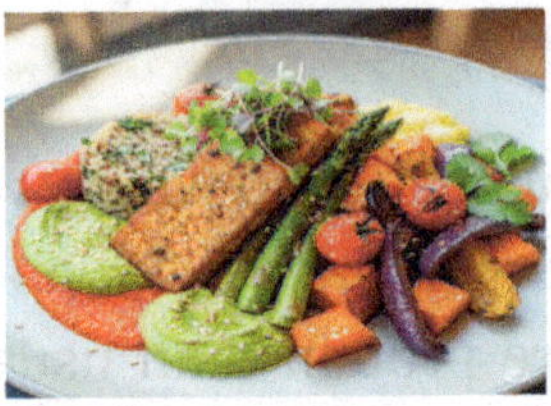

Adopting a new kidney is a fresh start. What you choose to eat plays an undeniably huge role in its long-term health and your overall well-being. Your diet as a not a restrictive chore.

Think of it as a powerful, proactive tool designed to protect your precious new organ and keep you feeling your best.

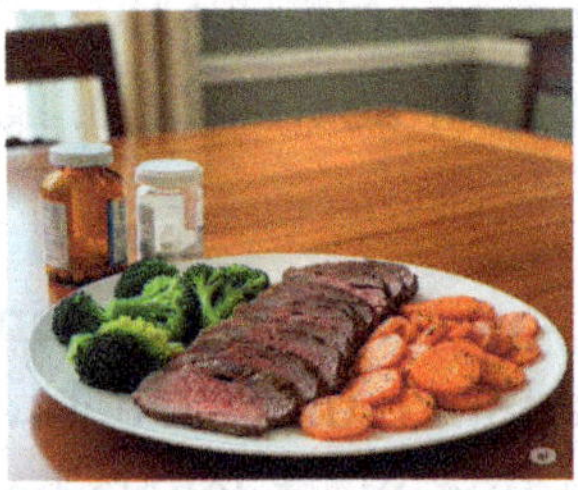

It's crucial to understand there isn't a "one-size-fits-all" diet plan after a transplant. Your personal eating strategy will be as unique as you are. Your dietary needs and choices should consider:

- **Your Unique Body:** Do you have co-existing conditions like diabetes, high blood pressure, or other specific health considerations that require tailored dietary approaches?
- **Your Medication "Cocktail":** The mix of powerful medications keeping your new kidney healthy is complex, and certain foods can significantly interfere with their effectiveness or even cause adverse reactions.
- **Your Personal Tastes & Lifestyle:** Eating should be an enjoyable experience! A sustainable diet is one that you can stick with, incorporating foods you genuinely like within the necessary guidelines.

1.1.1 - Smart Choices / Smart Future

A dietitian can help you create meals that work for your taste buds, your cooking skills (or lack of them - I struggle with boiling water for pasta), and any special dietary needs you might have.

This isn't the time for fast-food or late-night pizza deliveries! Your kidney and immune system need fresh, balanced fuel, not a sodium and fat overload. Over time, you mis-nomatch some but in the early stages, focus on clean, nourishing meals.

Quick Tips:

- Aim for a protein source at each meal; talk to your dietitian about your target grams per day.
- Avoid high-sodium "restaurant-style" foods early—read labels if using packaged items.
- Keep meals simple: grilled or baked lean protein + soft cooked vegetables + a controlled carb (if appropriate).
- Cook in small batches and refrigerate/freeze safely to avoid temptation of risky takeout.
- Ask your dietitian for flavor boosters (herbs, safe spices) so food doesn't feel bland.
- Always practice food safety: wash hands, cook to proper temperatures, avoid raw or undercooked items.
- Avoid protein supplements / bars unless your dietitian has approved them. Some "health" foods, you would discover that it may be less healthy than you thought.

1.2 - Medications vs Your Menu: An Important Partnership

You're taking a vital "cocktail" of medications – primarily anti-rejection drugs – specifically designed to prevent your body from identifying your new kidney as a foreign invader. These drugs are truly medical miracles, offering you a second chance at life. But they are very particular about what they "mix" with in your system.

For instance, one of my prescriptions has serious, potentially dangerous interactions with foods like shellfish, starfruit, and grapefruit. (So, no more Greyhounds, Salty Dogs, or Sea Breezes when out with friends!) These aren't just minor interactions; consuming them with certain medications can lead to serious complications and interactions, potentially harming your new kidney or causing severe side effects.

Your transplant team, especially the dietitians and pharmacists, are your absolute go-to experts for specific details regarding these interactions. As new and improved anti-rejection medications become available (and medical science is constantly advancing!), each will come with its own unique list of foods, common herbs, or even dietary supplements to avoid.

The golden rule here is non-negotiable: Always, always know what your eating and ask for guidance if you are unsure! Your vigilance in this area is a critical part of protecting your health.

1.3 - Guarding Against Germs: Food Safety is Your Superpower

Infection is a top concern for all transplant patients. Your anti-rejection meds, while life-saving, work by calming your immune system. This weakens your defenses against everyday germs.

Effective food safety starts even before cooking, with diligent food handling practices. This includes:

- Thorough Hand Washing: Before, during, and after handling food.
- Sanitizing Counters and Cooking Surfaces.
- Cleaning Cooking Utensils before and after each use.
- Preventing Cross-Contamination: Keep raw meats separate from ready-to-eat foods (fruits and vegetables) especially when cooking/preparing. Use separate cutting boards and utensils for raw and cooked items.
- Cooking to Safe Temperatures: Use a digital food thermometer to ensure all foods their proper internal temperatures, killing harmful bacteria.
- Proper Chilling and Storage: Refrigerate perishable foods promptly. Never leave cooked food out at room temperature for more than two hours.

Mastering food safety habits reduce food borne illness.

1.4 - A few of the "avoid" items that commonly pose a risk:

- Deli sliced meats and cheeses: These can harbor Listeria, a nasty bacteria. Handle properly and reheat or even avoid them.
- Raw or undercooked beef, pork, fish, and poultry: No rare steaks, sushi, or runny yolks! All meats, poultry, and seafood must be cooked thoroughly to the recommended safe internal temperatures.
- Unpasteurized dairy products: This includes raw milk, unpasteurized cheeses (like some Brie, Camembert, Blue, or Feta, unless specifically labeled pasteurized), and unpasteurized juices or ciders.
- Raw or lightly cooked eggs: Avoid homemade mayonnaise, Caesar dressing, hollandaise sauce, or cookie dough made with raw eggs. Use pasteurized egg products if a recipe calls for raw egg.
- Raw sprouts: Alfalfa, clover, mung bean, or radish sprouts can be breeding grounds for bacteria.
- Buffet / salad bars: Foods sitting at room temperature can quickly become contaminated. Safer to just avoid.
- Untreated water: (More on this below!)
- Herbal supplements and "natural" remedies: Many of these can interact dangerously with your medications or directly harm your kidney. NEVER take any supplement without clearing it with your transplant team first.

1.5 - Water Wisdom: Your Everyday Hydration

One of the subjects that often comes up is the source of drinking water. Many people think "water is water is water." It is... and it isn't. While it looks clear, it can contain microscopic nasties that your immune system, now off duty to protect your new kidney, just isn't prepared to fight.

- **Country Well Water:** If you're on well water, it's especially vulnerable to viruses, bacteria (from septic systems or agricultural runoff), and hard minerals. Even if it looks clean, it can be a silent threat.

  If you are on a private well, many county health districts can provide information on water quality testing. I would still distill and / or filter regardless

- **City/Municipal Water:** Don't assume city water is always perfect from the tap. While treated at the plant, the journey through miles of pipes can be problematic. Old supply lines can have tiny cracks or loose fittings, allowing seepage of contaminants (like groundwater or even tree roots invading the pipe!) *after* the purification process.

  Yes, tree roots can find a little drip from a water line, leading to invasion of cracked areas.

1.5 - Water Cleaning Systems: Beyond Softening

When we talk about 'cleaning' water, we're not just referring to water softeners (which deal with mineral hardness). We're talking about systems that actively *clean* and *purify* water from invisible threats.

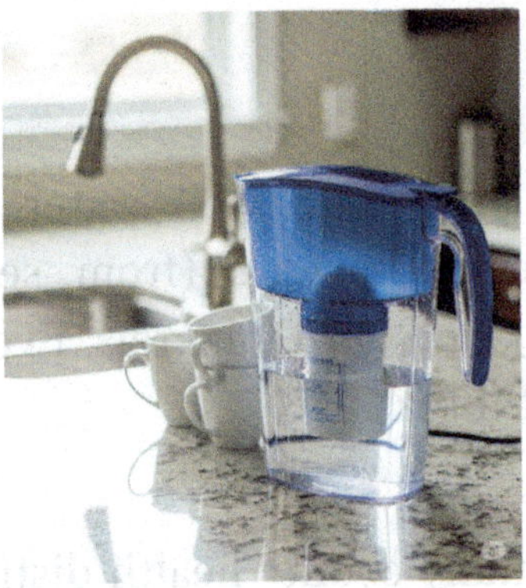

Water filter

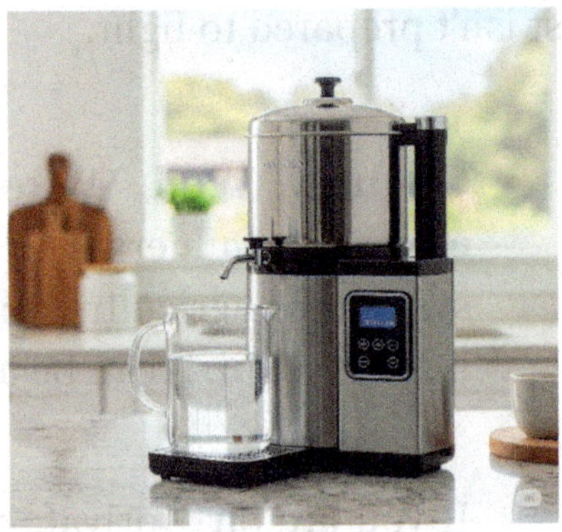

Distillation system

Your kidney is new, but is picky - and worth protecting

After my transplant, I was living in the country on a small farm. My water came from a private well—no filtration, no treatment, just straight from the ground. Some good friends chipped in and bought me a countertop water distiller. The well was never tested for microorganisms, but the amount of hard minerals—especially lime—was enough to raise eyebrows.

Later, I bought a house, moving into a city with municipal water, I kept using the distiller. And guess what? The buildup in the distiller's kettle got even worse. So much for "cleaner" city water.

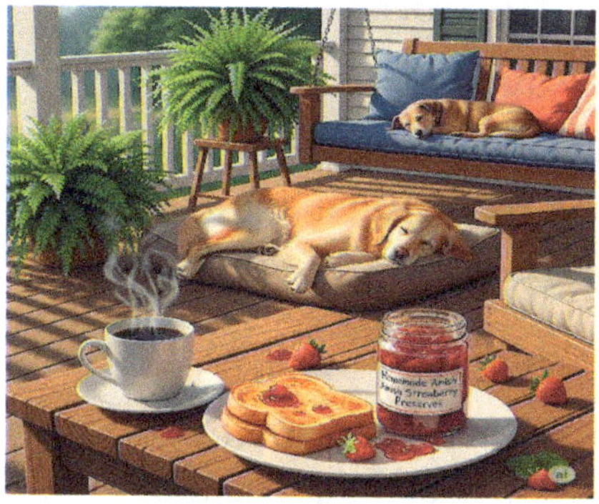

I use the distiller plus a two-stage carbon filter system. After distilling, I pour the water into the filter. This setup gives me easy access for water to make life-preserving coffee... and makes cooking a little safer too.

1.5.1 - Water Filtration:

- This is great for removing larger particles, sediment, chlorine, and some mineral deposits (like lime). Think of it like a very fine sieve.
- There's a huge variety of filters – from pitcher filters to faucet mounts to whole-house systems. Discussing the pros / cons is truly beyond this guide, but know they vary in what they can remove.
- A good multi-stage water filter system is a smart idea, especially if you rely on well water or if your home is far from the city water treatment plant. (Remember, older pipes were sometimes made with iron and lead, which can unfortunately leach into the water.)

1.5.2 - Water Distillation:

This is a fantastic way to get truly pure water. It involves heating water to a boiling point, turning it into steam. This steam is then collected and cooled back into a liquid state.

Two big benefits for transplant patients:

1.5.2.1 - Germ Killer: The boiling process effectively kills nearly all bacteria, viruses, and other microorganisms in the water.

1.5.2.1 - Mineral Remover: When the water turns to steam, most hard minerals, heavy metals, and other non-volatile contaminants (like nitrates or salts) are left behind in the chamber. This leaves nearly pure H2O.

1.5.2.1 - The PFAS Question: Ironically, there are some forms of chemicals ***not*** removed by distillation, most notably PFAS (Per- and Polyfluoroalkyl Substances). Before you call an attorney about "PFAS poisoning," understand that PFAS is an entire *class* of man-made chemicals used in countless everyday items like non-stick cookware, water-repellent fabrics, and firefighting foams. They are pervasive in the environment.

1.5.2.1 - Tackling PFAS: Certain specialized **three-stage filter systems** (mentioned above) with activated carbon may be more effective at reducing PFAS contaminants than distillation alone.

1.5.2.1 - The "Purest" Option: If you want the purest water possible, combining a good multi-stage filter (especially one targeting specific chemicals like PFAS) *and* distillation would be your best bet.

In case you're thinking distilling sounds a lot like how they make moonshine and whiskey, you're not wrong! The basic principle of separating liquids by boiling and condensing is the same.

(You'll have to do your own research on moonshining – though that might be a future book too. Feel free to contact me if you would like me to tackle that subject next.)

In Closing

Know and understand: The water you drink and cook with directly enters your body and, if contaminated, could introduce bacteria and viruses that your immune system is now less equipped to handle. Making informed choices about your water source is another way you actively protect your new kidney.

I was never a fan of tossing water bottles away – I would reuse them for weeks until they became soft and could possibly start leaking. I would refill from the sink. I now fill a sports bottle from a counter top water filter. I am getting clean water and not adding to the plastic waste in the landfill.

Chapter 2 - Sanitation Without Paranoia

Say hello to your new friends – paper towels, sanitizing wipes, bleach and anti-bacteria spray.

My transplant happened right at the start of the COVID-19 lockdowns and infection scares — so sanitation, already a critical concern for transplant patients, suddenly became a full-on lifestyle.

Somethings often recommended:

- sanitizing surfaces
- using gloves or hand sanitizer in public
- washing your hands like it's a part-time job
- Showering and changing clothes after being around large groups of people (think grocery stores, airports, or waiting rooms)

If you think about it, these should be normal practice anyway.

Now take all that... and multiply it by ten and you have life as a transplant recipient in the COVID 19 era.

2.1 - Sanitation as a Way of Life (Not a Panic Button)

They say cleanliness is next to godliness. For transplant patients, it's next to **a happy and healthy life!**

Right after surgery, you'll have an open wound — a literal hole in your body — which is basically an express lane for unwanted bacteria and viruses. Combine that with a weakened immune system thanks to anti-rejection medications, and cleanliness moves from optional to essential. And while I say this with all due respect to the naturally tidy among us, I've known more than a few germaphobes who'd feel right at home here.

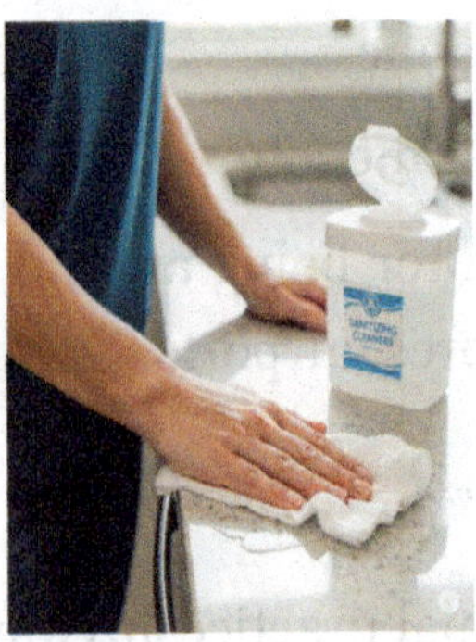

All the normal surfaces you clean anyway – counter tops, stove tops, refrigerator doors and handles, microwaves, kitchen appliances, kitchen sink and bathroom fixtures and more – will now get extra attention from you. Just remember: "Life's simple pleasures: a healthy kidney and a clean counter top."

Personally, I'm not big on having "strangers" in my house — and by strangers, I mean anyone who doesn't live here. (This includes random chainsaw-wielding hitchhikers in goalie masks). After any visitors leave, I give high-touch surfaces a quick wipe-down. It's not paranoia. It's just good practice.

2.2 - My Everyday Sanitation Kit

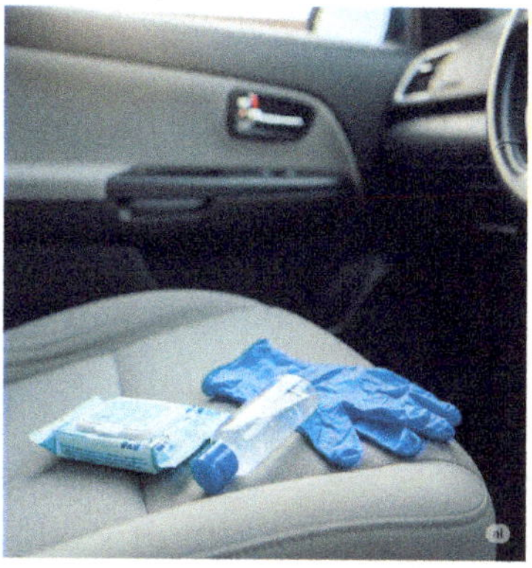

I keep a mini arsenal in both my car and RV:

1. Sanitizing wipes
2. Disposable gloves
3. Hand sanitizer

I use gloves at gas stations or ATMs, and I sanitize after shopping.

When flying, I pack several travel-sized sanitizing wipe packs – one for my carry-on and backups in my luggage. Before settling into my seat, I wipe down everything: armrests (top, bottom, and sides), headrest, tray table (front, back, and hinges), and the back of the seat in front of me. If you're thinking, "Wow, that's a lot," just remember the seat's last occupant could have had a cold, the flu, or something else entirely. Bonus tip: offer wipes to your seatmates – it's a great way to make friends or, at the very least, look like the most prepared person on the plane.

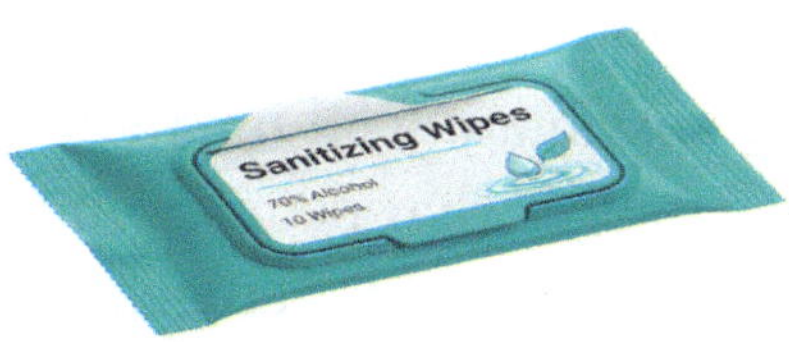

Forget AmEx, never leave home without your supply

2.3 - Eating Out (Without Freaking Out)

At restaurants, I'll often use a sanitizing wipe on the table. I also clean my hands after handling a menu that has been handled by who knows how many people. I bet you never thought about the number of people who handled salt & pepper, ketchup, mustard, hot sauce, etc. before you sat down at the table. You will never look at those on a restaurant's table the same way again.

At buffets, I sanitize my hands after picking up any shared utensils — because honestly, have you *seen* how many people handle those tongs in an hour?

(Before you scream at me because I said avoid buffets in other sections, I don't go very often, only on special occasions, like for example celebrating the Detroit Lions winning the Superbowl or the Seattle Mariners winning the World Series.)

I have had a few people I noticed {plus likely more I did not see} give me curious glances when I am cleaning utensils before using in a restaurant. You know what – I would rather increase my livability by reducing possible infections than give a hoot about what people think. Factually, what people think is seldom on my care list anyway. My health and well-being is my top priority.

2.4 - A Little Effort Goes a Long Way

I have never had many issues with colds and the like. Sure, the occasional bug sneaks through, but it was always rare. Now, with my immune system dialed way down, I'm even more serious about avoiding exposure — not in a bubble-boy kind of way, but definitely not living carelessly either. COVID is still out there, the flu makes annual visits and random viruses are like dandelions blowing in the wind.

Have you ever noticed most people grab the top of door handles when opening them at stores, restaurants and businesses. Once you think about that, you will likely more often reach to a lesser used area and casually wipe your hand after you are inside. I catch myself wiping my hand on my shirt out of habit. It may not be perfectly clean – but cleaner than the door handle.

When exiting, I am more likely to lean into the door rather than use my hand to place on the same spot the last 50 people used to push open the door. You could say, I've mastered the art of the 'no-touch' door exit, shouldering or backing my way out. It's like a secret handshake for the hygienically aware.

2.5 - Grocery Hacks & Germ-Blocking Tips

During COVID, one of my hacks: only bring perishable items into the house right away. If the weather allows, leave dry goods or non-essentials in the car for a day or two. While it may not kill everything, every bit helps — and sometimes one less germ really is just that: one less. You can think like a reverse lottery - the one germ you block might have been the one with your number on it.

As for reusable shopping bags — yes, they're great for the environment, but they're also germ hotels if not cleaned regularly. After each use, wash them in warm or hot water with a non-bleach disinfectant (check the label to avoid ruining them).

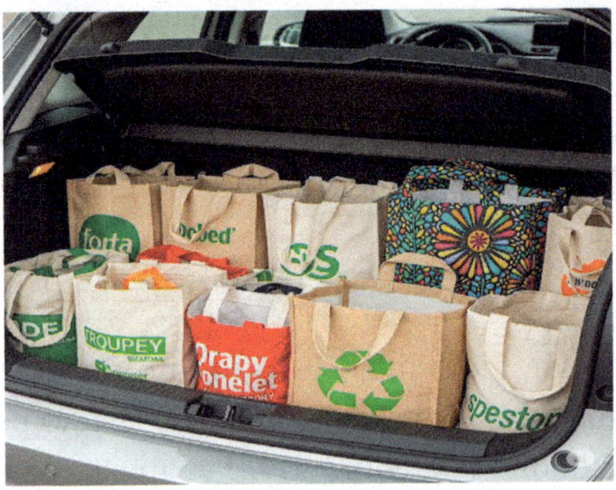

And here's an extra tip: don't bring bags in the store. Load groceries directly into the cart, then transfer to your bags at the car. The bags are in or on your cart and it ain't clean — unless you're the one doing it.

In Plain Language

You don't need to live in fear – just live like Grandma taught you.

And she wasn't wrong. Good ol' common sense goes a long way. Wash your hands like you were taught as a youngin'. Wipe down your counters like company's comin'. Treat that raw meat like it's got a grudge against your gut. Scrub your veggies like they rolled through the garden twice. And for heaven's sake, don't eat anything that smells like it could walk off the plate on its own.

Grandma always said, *"Soap, sunshine, and common sense'll fix more than folks realize."*

Keeping your head on straight, your habits clean, and be mindful of your surroundings – no need to wrap yourself in bubble wrap.

You might find this closing corny, but after discussing all the problems with being safe, I wanted to pick you up a little. I hope you smiled just a little.

Chapter 3 - Getting Out There After Transplant

Congratulations! You're officially out of the dialysis dungeon and back in the world with a fresh passport to freedom. But pump the brakes before you start booking zipline tours or decide it's time to summit Kilimanjaro,—this isn't

Kidney Quest: The Kidney Comeback World Tour.

Think of it like downloading a new app: it looks great, but you still need to run updates, adjust the settings, and maybe charge your battery first.

Your body just went through major surgery, and while your spirit might be ready for adventure, your stamina might still be on the couch asking for one more nap.

Start small. A leisurely lap at the school track is a perfect start. Regain your strength one step at a time (literally). Maybe you hiked 3 trails like a champ, great! But for now, let's not pretend that walking through Costco on a Saturday isn't already its own endurance challenge.

What follows are some tips to help you pace yourself without losing that sense of excitement. It's your comeback tour.

3.1 - Ease Back In Gradually:

Start with small and gradually increase your exposure to larger activities. This helps you adjust without feeling overwhelmed.

3.2 - Prioritize Hand Hygiene:

Frequent and thorough handwashing is one of the most effective ways to prevent infection. Carry hand sanitizer with you for times when soap and water aren't available

3.3 - Be Mindful of Your Health:

Pay attention to how you're feeling. If you're tired, run-down, or starting to feel sick, best to cancel plans and rest.

3.4 - Communicate with Your Team:

Always discuss your travel and social plans with your transplant team. They can provide specific recommendations, vaccinations, and other precautions based on your individual health status.

3.5 - Vaccinations and Medications:

Ensure you are up-to-date on all recommended vaccinations. When traveling, pack extra medication in case of delays.

3.6 - Sun Protection:

Transplant medications can make your skin more sensitive to the sun. Use a high-SPF sunscreen, wear protective clothing, and seek shade to prevent sunburn.

3.7 - Food and Water Safety:

Be cautious about what you eat and drink, especially when traveling. Avoid raw or under-cooked foods and stick to bottled water to minimize the risk of foodborne illness.

3.8 - Setting Boundaries:

It's okay to say no to social invitations that make you uncomfortable or feel risky. You are in control of your own health and well-being.

(Don't try this excuse to get out of Thanksgiving Dinner at your in-laws house. Also, don't ask how I know.)

3.9 - Support System:

Lean on your friends, family, and support groups. They can provide encouragement, understanding, and a safe space to share your experiences as you reintegrate into social life. Especially initially, you will want the buddy system - someone else with you in case you get tired, weak or face issues.

3.10 - What are your plans with your freedoms from dialysis?

That international trip you always wanted, A six state motorcycle tour? Two weeks camping? Out of state family reunions you skipped in the past? You have been given the gift of life - start living it again.

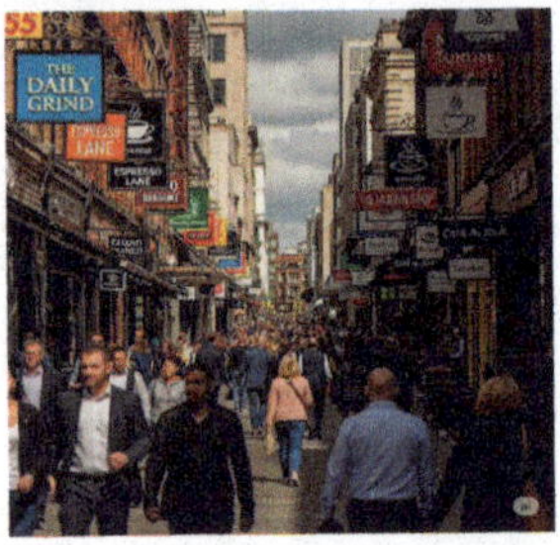

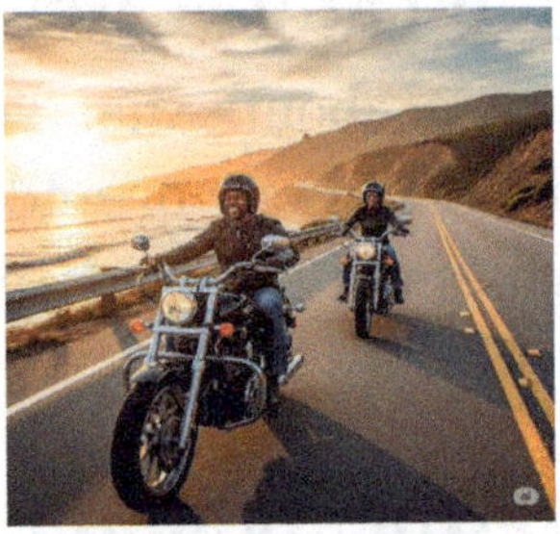

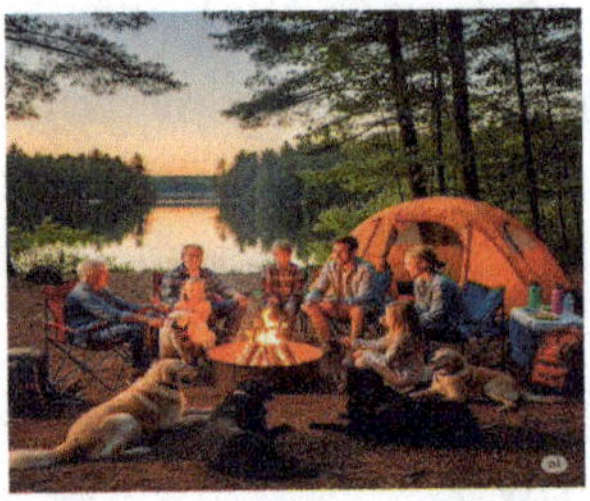

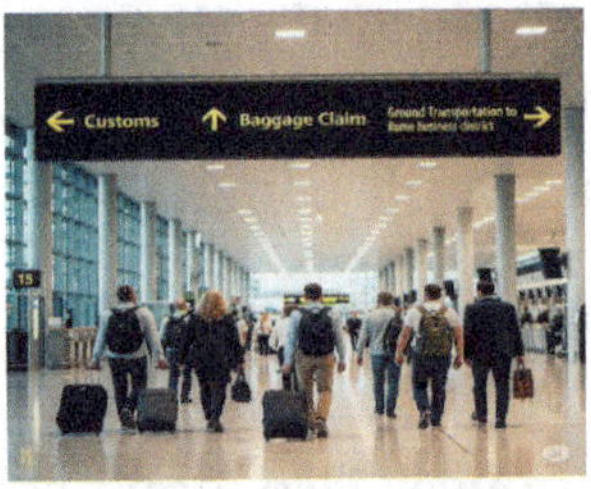

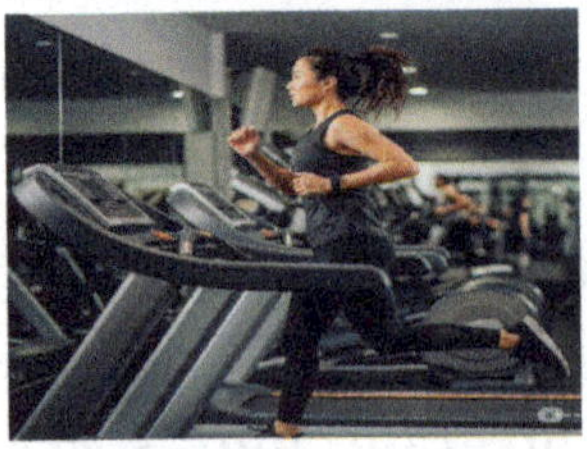

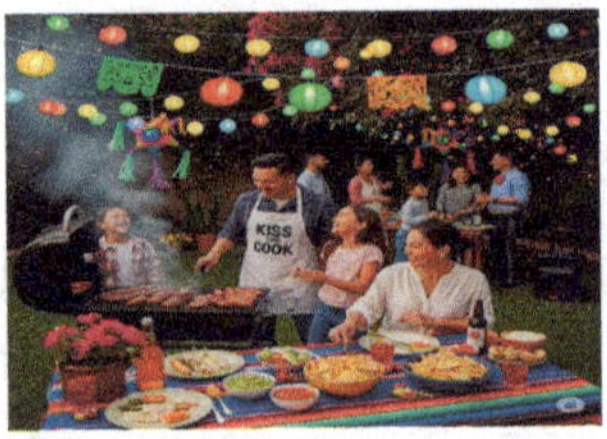

Chapter 4 - Helping Others While Helping Yourself

Survival is courage. Sharing what you survived is strength.

You've made it through transplant surgery, the meds haven't turned you into a gremlin, and your doctor hasn't had to hide your chart behind a sigh. That's progress. Now what?

Believe it or not, one of the best ways to continue your own healing is by lifting up someone else. Weird, right? But science backs it up—helping others improves your mood, sense of purpose, and (bonus) can even reduce stress. It's like a gym for your soul, except the only membership fee is your time and willingness to show up.

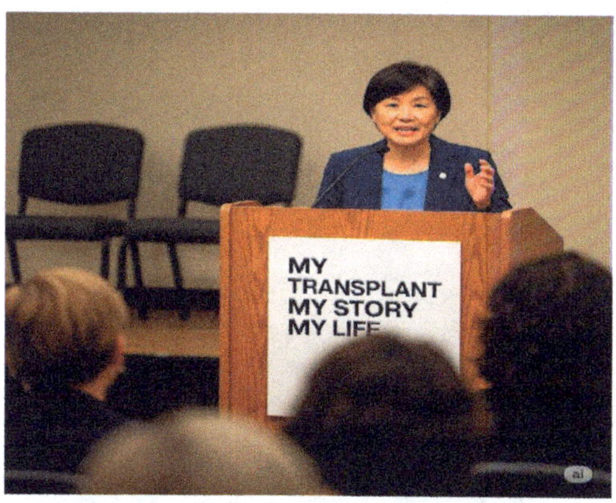

Whether you want to dip a toe in or dive headfirst, here are a few ways you can pay it forward without draining your new kidney's goodwill account.

4.1 - Volunteering: No Cape Required

You don't need to rebuild houses or teach yoga to seniors (unless that's your thing). Sometimes, just helping out at a community event or offering an extra hand at your transplant center's next info night is enough. Remember, just showing people you *made it through* speaks volumes.

Many hospitals have volunteering positions for a variety of purposes and goals. These can be even more critical at small local hospitals that run on thinner budgets than the mega medical hubs.

These could be positions running the gift shop, an information desk, a book cart (taking loaner books to patients), assisting with fund raising events or at health out reach events.

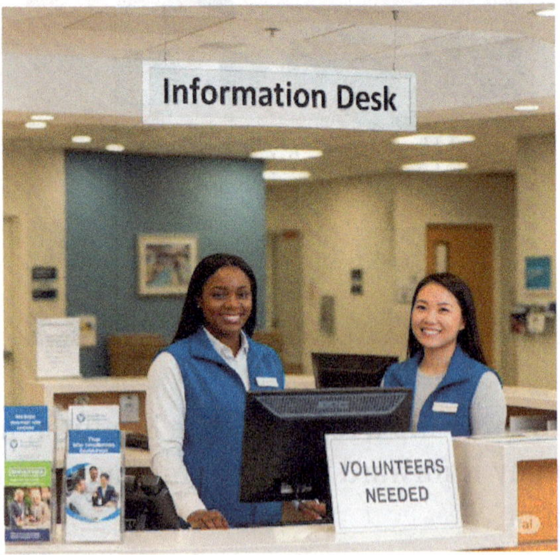

Before my transplant, I was volunteering in the snack bar one day a week for a small (only 22 beds!!!) hospital.

After the transplant, it was COVID era so I never returned because of new hospital policies and my limitations because of the transplant drugs.

I was actually at the snack bar when I got the pre-notice call of a possible transplant. The come now call was later that night.

4.2 - Counseling: You're Not a Therapist, But You *Are* a Survivor

You know things most people don't know —like what hospital pudding *really* tastes like or why nurses wake you up to offer you a sleeping pill. By offering perspective and encouragement to someone diagnosed with kidney failure can be powerful. Like tossing a rope to someone in the hole you climbed out of.

You're not a licensed counselor — and no one's expecting you to be. But being a shoulder to cry on or just someone who listens can make a big difference. Sometimes folks just need to vent, and once they do, they're ready to help themselves. If they need more help, your support might be what gives them the push to talk to a pro. In a country where therapy still feels like a taboo, your voice might be the one that helps break that stigma.

4.4 - Support Groups: Therapy With Snacks

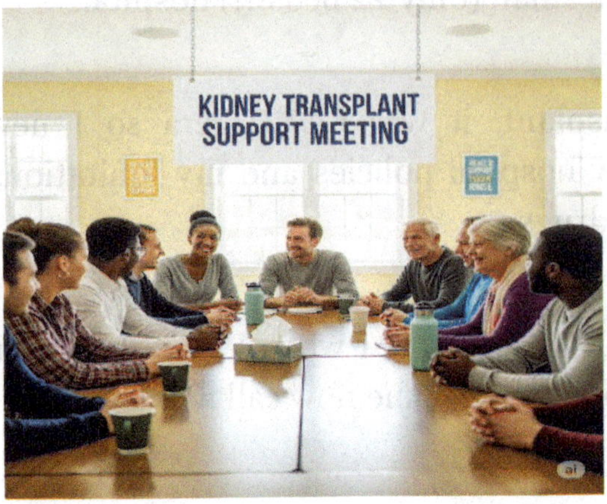

Whether virtual or in-person, support groups offer the chance to be both the one who listens *and* the one who's heard. You might even make real friends, not just the kind who say "Let me know if you need anything" and then vanish faster than donuts at the police department's morning meetings.

4.3 - Buddy Systems: Healing in Pairs (Or More)

Having a "kidney buddy" is underrated. You get someone who speaks your language: meds, labs, fatigue, awkward belly scars, and all. You help each other stay accountable, vent safely, and maybe even laugh through the "Did I just forget what day it is again?" moments.

Wrap-Up: You've Got This (And Maybe a Muffin, Too)

Look, you don't have to be a superhero in scrubs or start a nationwide foundation. If all you ever do is show up once a month, coffee in hand, to say "Yep, I've been there too".

Congratulations – you're officially making the world a better place.

Helping others while healing yourself isn't about big speeches or perfectly timed wisdom. It's about being real. And after everything you've been through, *real* is your superpower.

So go ahead – be someone's calm in the storm, their "I get it," their proof life after transplant is not just possible... it's worth it.

And hey, if snacks are involved, even better.

Chapter 5 - Support Groups online

(Even If You Still Think "Zoom" Means Fast)

Support groups come in all flavors — in-person, online, social media-based, or sometimes just two folks on folding chairs with a shared story and a coffee thermos. The key is finding a group that feels like a fit, not a chore. Because let's face it, you've had enough appointments already.

5.1 - If You're Tech-Savvy (or Know a Grandkid Who Is):

5.1.1 - Facebook: It's still the town square for kidney groups. Search terms like *"kidney transplant support," "dialysis warriors,"* or *"transplant life."*

5.1.2 - Reddit: Surprisingly decent. Try r/KidneyTransplant or r/Dialysis.

5.1.3 - Zoom/Meetup: Virtual groups hosted by hospitals, nonprofits, or patient-led groups. Bonus: You can attend in pajama pants and no one knows.

Protip: You may or may not be wearing pajama pants - but {pajama} tops are strenuously encouraged.

5.2 - If You Prefer Analog or Low-Tech:

5.2.1 - Ask Your Transplant Center: Many hospitals have peer mentor programs or know of nearby support meetings (some even have potlucks, just sayin').

5.2.2 - Libraries, Churches & Community Centers: They may already host health-related gatherings or are willing to start one if there is enough interest.

5.2.3 - Your Local Coffee Shop Bulletin Board: Old-school? Yes. Effective? Sometimes surprisingly so.

5.3 Where to Find Support Groups (Without Needing a Tech Degree)

I have no experiences with these groups and can not personally endorse any of them. Try 2 or 3 and pick the one you most connect with.

5.3.1 - National Kidney Foundation

https://www.kidney.org
Look for their "Peer Mentoring" and "NKF Peers" programs. They'll match you with someone who's been through what you're going through — kind of like a transplant pen pal who *gets it.*

5.3.2 - American Association of Kidney Patients (AAKP)

https://aakp.org
Offers webinars, patient meetups, ambassador programs, and even an advocacy group if you feel like putting your cape on.

5.3.3 - Renal Support Network (RSN)

https://www.rsnhope.org
Started by a kidney transplant recipient, they offer virtual support groups, podcasts, and patient stories with just the right mix of heart and humor.

5.3.4 - Transplant Recipients International Organization (TRIO)

https://www.trioweb.org

Open to all organ transplant patients, with chapters and virtual meetings. Serious topics, but a welcoming vibe.

5.3.5 - MyTransplantLife

https://mytransplantlife.com

A growing online hub of blogs, community events, and resources built specifically for post-transplant life.

5.3.6 HealthUnlocked – Kidney Community

https://healthunlocked.com/kidneysupport

Free to join, kind of like a kidney-focused forum where you can post questions or just lurk and learn. Not flashy, but genuinely helpful.

5.3.7 - Dialysis Patient Citizens (DPC)

https://www.dialysispatients.org

Great for pre-transplant patients or those navigating dialysis and the transplant process. Offers education, policy involvement, and community.

5.4 Offline Ideas (Just as Powerful):

5.4.1 - Ask your transplant center or clinic social worker if they list of support groups or mentor programs.

5.4.2 - Local churches, YMCAs, senior centers, or veterans' organizations often host health-related group meetups — some just need a nudge to start one.

5.4.2 - If all else fails, try this line on a neighbor:
"Know anyone else with a recycled kidney? I'm starting a club and we've got coffee."

Bottom line: You don't have to do this alone. Whether you're venting, laughing, or asking if it's normal for your meds to make your eyebrows grow faster than your hair — someone out there *gets it*.

And if you don't find the right group? Start your own. You've earned the title of Kidney Comeback Captain.

V. Closing Thoughts:

Hang On and Enjoy the Ride

I was so accustomed to dialysis and its routine that I never let my mind imagine anything different. I felt buried in a pit with walls so high there was no way out. *This is it,* I told myself. *This is what life will be.* I reminisced about the past. I refused to dream about the future.

Then one day, I looked at those walls and realized they were closing in. That was my wake-up call. I was too young and had too much to offer — to others and to myself — to let the walls win. I started looking for the tools to dig my way out.

Looking back now, my kidney transplant journey felt a lot like riding the Millennium Force roller coaster at Cedar Point. (Unpaid plug — but Cedar Point, I'm available!)

The climb started slow — *click, click, click* — with every doctor visit, lab test, and transplant team meeting. I wasn't sure I'd ever make it to the top. But I kept climbing, because I wanted to see what was on the other side.

Then, out of nowhere – WHOOSH – I was flying downhill: surgery, recovery, meds, more meds, side effects, and an endless parade of doctors, nurses, and specialists. The car was moving so fast there was no getting off, even if I wanted to.

There were moments I was upside down, twisting through dark tunnels like a demented Universal Studios [also unpaid plug, call me ;)] horror ride. I'd see a light ahead, thinking the tunnel was ending – only to find it was a fire-breathing dragon. A setback. Something didn't go as planned. But instead of panicking, I stayed on the ride, trusting the process and the people helping me.

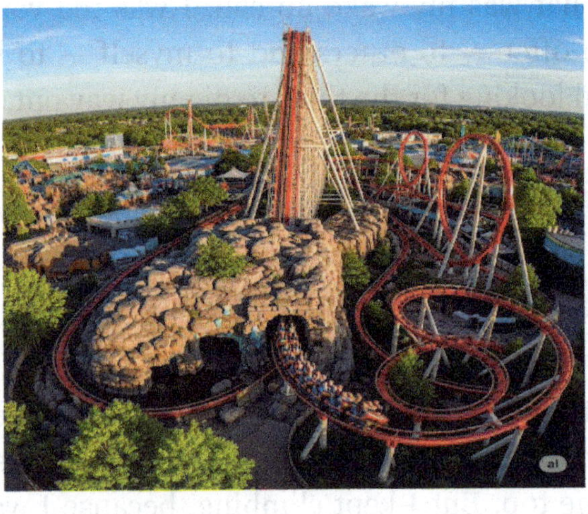

As suddenly as the tunnel began, it ended – but then came the corkscrews. Ups, downs, spirals. At times I felt like a coin flipping in midair, not knowing how I'd land.

And then, finally, the ride began to level out. The wind was still in my face, but I wasn't holding on for dear life anymore. I was riding it. Living. Breathing. Healing.

Finally ... it was over. I was on to new things, new places, new people, new experiences.

Maybe you've already started the process, or maybe you're just thinking about getting in line for the transplant roller coaster. Either way, it's okay to be nervous. I sure was. I didn't have it all figured out. I was scared, broke, tired, and unsure. I didn't know if I was more afraid of dying... or of living.

But here's the thing – you're going to meet angels in sneakers: doctors, nurses, transplant coordinators who will know your body better than you do. Lean on them. Trust them. Ask them questions. They're there for more than scribbling prescriptions.

You'll learn more about insurance, financial and legal matters than you ever wanted to know. It's not easy, but help exists: organizations, crowdfunding, support groups and tools that let you seek help without feeling like you're begging on a street corner.

I might have chosen transplant sooner if I'd known my options – I want you to explore and know yours.

And don't forget your mental health. This isn't just a physical ride – it's a mental one. Even the strongest people need someone to talk to. If the load feels heavy, ask for help. There's no shame in it.

When the dust settles and your new life begins, live it. Go outside. Sit in the sun. Hug your people. Eat a taco. Pet a dog. Eat another taco. Pet another dog. Smell the flowers - unless you have allergies. Find joy in the ordinary. You've earned it.

When you and your support team step off the transplant roller coaster, your legs will be steady in a way they haven't been in years. Behind you, the steel tracks twist and loop against the sky, but the rumble of the ride is fading.

A warm breeze carries the scent of funnel cakes, corn dogs and popcorn. You pass the snack stand without stopping. Now is not the time for comfort food - it's time for charting new horizons and stepping boldly into whatever adventure waits beyond the gates.

Up ahead, bathed in afternoon sunlight, stands a tall signpost of polished oak and brass:
Left: The Train – Next Stop: New Adventures.
Straight Ahead: The Open Road – Miles of Possibilities.
Right: Flights – International & Domestic.

Each path calls to you. To the left, shining rails stretch toward rolling hills and open sky. Straight ahead, a highway winds through golden valleys toward distant towns. To the right, the air hums with jet engines as silver planes lift into the blue.

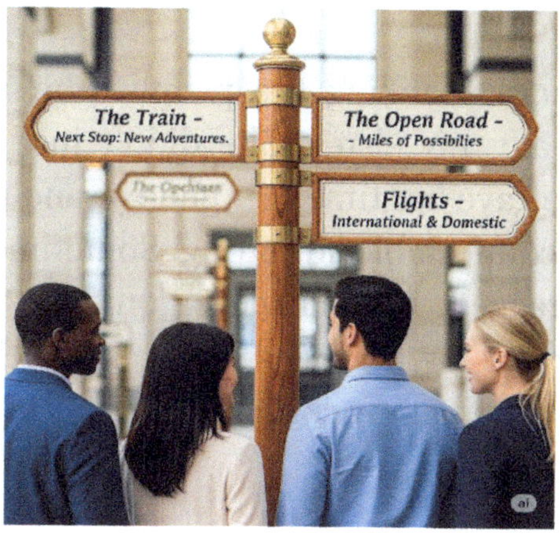

Which adventure will you pick first? Write it down. Look at it first thing each day and before you go to bed. Each time you read it, visualize it. This is more powerful than you think.

You stand there for a moment, taking it in — the colors sharper, the air richer, the ground solid beneath your feet. For the first time in a long time, you're not strapped into a ride someone else controls.

And buddy... it's worth every twist and turn.

You won't just have survived something hard – you'll have chosen to fight. You may not have had a choice in needing a transplant, but you *do* have a choice in how you face it. Hand over your ticket — the ride is ready to start. The rest of your life is waiting.

I can't close without thanking the people who made my ride possible – especially my sister. She didn't just show up; she outperformed. She gave her time, her energy, and probably more money than she's comfortable admitting. Sometimes she pushed, sometimes she dragged, but she never quit on me. Family – whether by blood or by choice – can make the impossible survivable. I had several in my corner.

— John Carter

VI. Appendixes - Extra Tools, More Ideas and Expanding Options

This final section offers bonus insights and resources that don't always fit into neat medical charts or transplant timelines – but matter just as much. These pages are here for reference, inspiration, and empowerment.

Appendixes in this section:

1. **My Story in Summary**
2. **Bio-Artificial Kidneys and The Future**
3. **Fundraising Without Feeling Like a Burden**
4. **Tips for Writing Request Letters**
5. **Being A Living Donor**
6. **Transferring to a New Transplant Center**

Appendix 1 - My Story In Summary

Earlier, I shared how I ended up on hemodialysis and gave glimpses of my transplant journey including getting "The Call," the hospital stay, surgery, and what followed. Now we go deeper. This is the honest look at life after transplant. It's not to scare you—it's to show you that while it's tough, it's absolutely doable.

A1.1 - The Transplant and Recovery

I had my kidney transplant at University of Michigan's – Ann Arbor Taubman Transplant Center. If you've ever wondered what it's like to recover from major surgery *during the start of a global pandemic*, well... let me take you there.

My surgery started at 2:00 PM on Friday, March 13, 2020. Yes, *Friday the 13th.* And yes, *the Friday COVID shut down Michigan.* While I was busy getting a brand-new kidney, the Governor of Michigan was busy locking down the state. As far as I know, mine was the last transplant performed for a while. If not the last one of the last few. I really slid in under the wire.

Because of fluid buildup from surgery, a spike in potassium, and all the extra meds in my system, I went straight from post-op to —you guessed it—*dialysis.* Yep, brand-new kidney and all, but the little guy hadn't punched the time clock yet. I didn't make it to my recovery room until almost midnight.

Saturday was pretty uneventful unless you count pain, exhaustion, and a heroic attempt at a hallway walk. I made it maybe one room down the hall before I turned to the nurse and said, "Yeah... this is far enough."

Sunday: rinse and repeat—but with another dialysis session. The kidney was still on vacation. Monday was the same. I got another round of dialysis and by late that night, they discharged me. My sister drove me two hours home through Michigan construction zones in the dark without a single complaint. Tuesday was mostly a fog of sleep, and pain meds.

By Wednesday, I was back at my dialysis clinic. Normally I used a county ride service. But with a fresh surgical wound and, you know, the global pandemic, my sister chauffeured me. She also drove me four more hours on Thursday for a post-op check-up in Ann Arbor. Friday, it was back to dialysis again. Glamorous, right?

I'm not telling you all this to bore you—though I'll admit, it's not exactly a summer blockbuster plot. I want you to see what a real recovery timeline can look like. There's no dramatic "happily ever after" on Day 3. There's just progress—slow, steady, real.

The following week brought home care nurses, blood draws, wound checks, more dialysis, and a biopsy. And then... something started to change.

A1.2 - The kidney had clocked in.

On March 26, I had the sudden, overwhelming urge to pee—but couldn't. I was literally in the bathroom every 30 minutes with no relief. In tears, I asked my sister to drive me to the ER.

Turns out, my bladder was full. Once they inserted a catheter, everything started flowing.

From that moment on the 26th, no more dialysis. The new kidney had finally decided it was time to get to work—and it didn't mess around.

Over the next weeks, I had follow-ups, another surgery (infection cleanup), with a short hospital stay. They started me the wound vac and discharged me. The wound vac was used until late May. It was always cared for by a home-care nurse.

Later I was switched wet-to-dry dressings twice a day—every day. My sister, with her lifetime of mom, grandma, and decades of Girl Scout experience, handled it like a pro.

There were months of healing, more visits to Ann Arbor. Labs at the local hospital. Home visits. It was routine without being routine.

A1.3 - Re-hospitalized - Staphylococcus aureus bacteria

A staph infection in December that landed me back in the hospital for Christmas. (My stocking was a hospital gown, and I do not recommend it.) After a couple of weeks in a rehab facility I was discharged on January 2, 2021.

Eventually, after wound clinics and antibiotics and more home health visits than I can count, I was released from all wound care by May 2021.

It was a year of setbacks, progress, more setbacks, and hard-earned victories.

But here's the deal: **I made it.**

And I'm here writing this because I want *you* to know that you can make it too. Not because you have to be strong all the time, but because this journey is about persistence, support, and giving yourself room to heal.

I broke down sometimes. I had days where I was scared, frustrated, or just plain tired of being tired. But I never gave up. And if I could fight my way through that year of hearling—you absolutely can too.

A1.4 - Me Today

Since my transplant in 2020, I've been living again.

I've regained 27 hours a week of *my* time. You might wonder, "Isn't dialysis only four hours three times a week?" Technically, yes—but the reality adds up fast.

Each session took 4 hours, plus 30 minutes before to get checked in and ready, and another 30 minutes afterward to recover before heading home. That's 5 hours already. Then there's the hour before, just to get up, get dressed, and get to the clinic. That's 6 hours.

By the time I got back home, I often needed a 3-hour nap just to feel human again. Six plus three equals nine hours, three times a week—27 hours gone. And I did not even include travel to get back to the house.

But now, those 27 plus hours are mine again. Mine to spend living, not existing. That's what this new kidney gave me—time, energy, and a second shot at life.

I've attended family reunions. I bought a house, moving to my own place. I worked GIG apps without having to think about dialysis treatments or plan my entire day around a machine.

For about a year, I volunteered as a Military Honor Guard honoring our Veterans— because I had the time and freedom to give. I have chatted on Facebook with people who have asked questions about getting a transplant. Again - without dialysis I can be online anytime 24/7 if someone needs to talk.

I've traveled — twice internationally to Thailand — without the stress of coordinating treatments along the way. {Actually it would have been impossible to do!!!} Each trip, from walking out the door to catch my flight to walking back in nearly four weeks later, was uninterrupted by medical treatments.

That kind of freedom is priceless. More travel is on the horizon — both across the U.S. and overseas. I have energy again. I have purpose. I have freedom.

I remain mindful of my labs, drawn at least every other month. But now, they're just part of the schedule — not **the** schedule. I can schedule my labs any day of the week convenient for me.

The main logistical constraint is receiving my transplant meds in person each month. So when I travel, I simply plan around my delivery dates. It's a small adjustment for a huge return.

I am no longer constrained by the clock - the alarm clock specifically. You know, the alarm that wakes you up at a certain time three days a week so you can get ready to leave for dialysis?

In short, I can once again take random day trips, enjoy weekends away, work, volunteer, and explore life on my own terms. While there are still dietary restrictions — and some foods that clash with my immunosuppressants — they're nothing like the limitations I faced on dialysis. Dairy Queen malts and takeout pizza, for example, are no longer on the banned list. I would prefer you keep this secret away from my dietitian.

Life isn't perfect — but it's *life* again. And that's everything.

Appendix 2 - Bio-artificial Kidneys And The Future

Disclaimer: Science is moving so fast, so fast your coffee might be cold before info released today is outdated. While I've done my best to share what's current, bio and artificial kidney research changes quicker than Uncle Earl's stories at a family reunion. So treat this as a friendly intro, not gospel. Always double-check the latest with real experts, research centers, or someone with a lab coat and not just a blog.

A2.1 - Implantable Bioartificial Kidneys (The Kidney Project - UCSF)

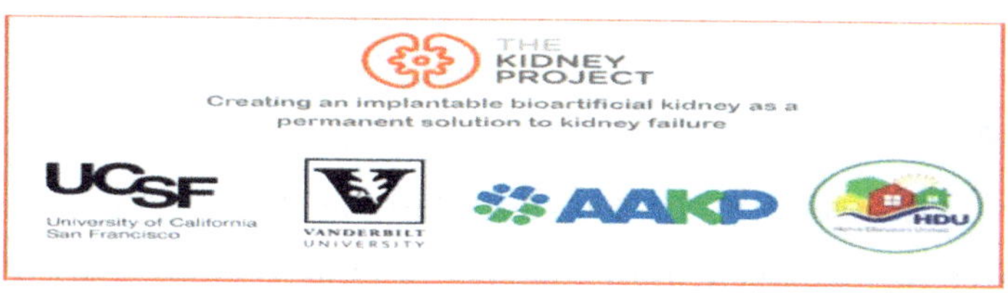

A national research and development collaboration based at the University of California, San Francisco (UCSF), The Kidney Project is working to create the first-ever surgically implantable bioartificial kidney. They are aiming for it to size of a coffee cup and operate without the need for an external power source. The goal is a permanent solution for kidney failure that would free patients from dialysis and the long wait for a human transplant, as well as the lifelong need for anti-rejection drugs.

The Kidney Project at UCSF is a leading effort developing a small, surgically implanted device with two main components:

A2.1.1 - Hemofilter: This part uses advanced silicon nanotechnology to filter blood, similar to the glomeruli in natural kidneys. It's designed to be powered by the patient's own blood pressure, eliminating the need for external pumps or power.

A2.1.2 - Bioreactor: This contains living human kidney cells that perform the biological functions of a kidney (reabsorbing essential nutrients, balancing electrolytes, producing hormones, etc.). The design aims to protect these cells from the body's immune system, potentially eliminating the need for immunosuppressant drugs.

Current Status:

They have successfully tested small-scale prototypes of both components in animals, demonstrating that they work together as intended. The biggest hurdle remains scaling up the device to a size and capacity suitable for human implantation and ensuring long-term functionality without clotting or issues.

Currently they estimate they are about 4-5 years away from being ready for human clinical trials, but this depends significantly on securing sufficient funding. Their ultimate goal is clinical trials by the end of the decade (2030). Commercialization could be by 2040 or before.

A2.2 - Wearable Artificial Kidneys (WAK)

While not fully implantable, these aim to free patients from the large, stationary dialysis machines.

Current Status: Several prototypes exist, like the Wearable Artificial Kidney (WAK) developed by Dr. Victor Gura's team. It's a miniaturized dialysis machine that can be worn, offering more flexibility.

The WAK has undergone human studies with promising results, but it's still experimental and not yet FDA approved for public use.

Other portable and desktop-sized devices are also in development, often focusing on dialysate regeneration to significantly reduce water usage, making them more practical for home or portable use.

A2.3 - Kidney Regeneration/Organoids

This is a more long-term, purely biological approach where researchers are working to grow kidney tissue or even whole kidneys in the lab using stem cells.

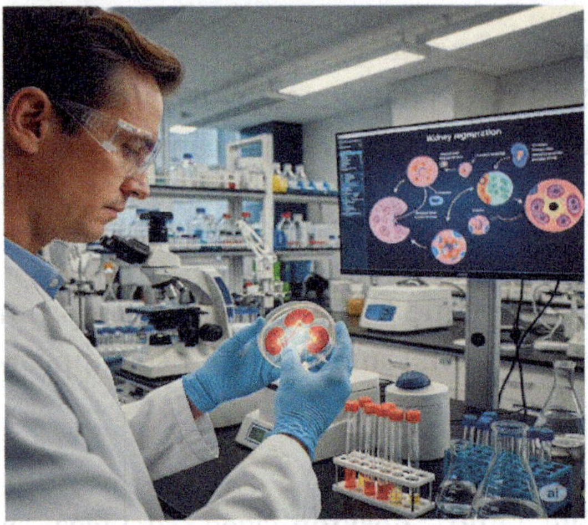

Current Status: Significant breakthroughs have occurred in creating kidney organoids (small, self-organized 3D cell cultures that mimic kidney structure and function). Researchers have even successfully grown nephrons (the filtering units of the kidney) in the lab and implanted them into mice.

This field is still in its early stages, but it holds immense promise for the future, potentially eliminating rejection issues if grown from a patient's own cells.

A2.4 - AI: The Hope For The future:

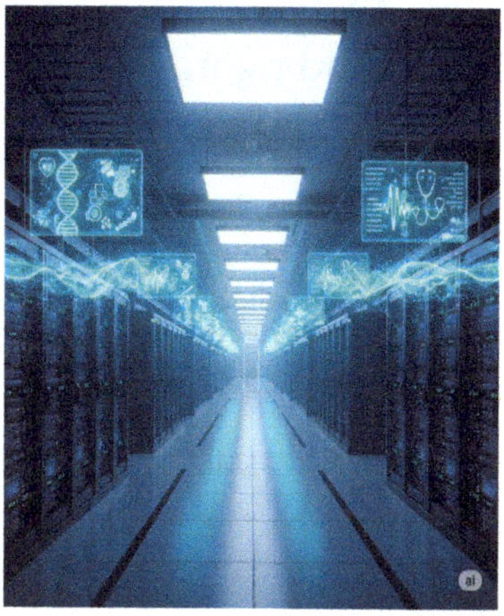

The potential role of AI. AI, machine learning, and advanced computational modeling are indeed poised to accelerate these timelines in several crucial ways:

- AI analyzes complex lab data, spots patterns, and helps design experiments to speed up development.
- AI rapidly scans existing drug data to find candidates that may slow kidney disease, ease complications, or support artificial organ function.
- AI models new biocompatible materials for implants that minimize clotting and immune reactions.
- AI tailors dialysis plans, predicts complications, and boosts performance of wearable kidney technology.
- AI improves trial design by finding ideal participants, predicting responses, shortening timelines, and sort results into valuable reports in minutes vs days.

It's exciting to think about how these powerful tools could genuinely shorten the path from lab to patient for something as transformative as an artificial kidney.

A2.4 - Why the "10 years" often stretches

A2.4.1 - Regulatory and Approval Process: The FDA approval process for medical devices is long and rigorous – as it should be. Devices must meet strict safety, reliability, and long-term durability standards.

A2.4.2 - Biocompatibility and Immune Response: Getting the body to accept and not attack or reject a device is a major hurdle. Materials must be completely biocompatible, resist clotting, and not trigger inflammation.

A2.4.3 - Miniaturization and Power Supply: Shrinking the technology small enough to be implantable or wearable – while still being powerful and efficient is a massive engineering challenge. These devices must run on minimal power without needing frequent charging or battery replacement.

A2.4.4 - Anti-Clotting and Filtering Efficiency: Artificial kidneys need to filter blood like the real thing, without causing clotting or needing constant blood thinners (which increase other medical risks). This is a delicate balancing act.

A2.4.5 - Clinical Trial Participation: Many advanced devices may stall because of a lack of suitable or willing participants for trials. Patients may fear the risks, or clinicians may hesitate to enroll them in something so experimental – especially when dialysis, as imperfect as it is, still works.

A2.4.6 - Healthcare System Adoption: Even after successful trials, convincing large healthcare systems and insurers to adopt and pay for new tech takes time. Widespread rollout requires building partnerships, retraining staff, updating billing codes, and lots of paperwork.

In Closing:

Developing a fully functional artificial kidney is one of medical science's most ambitious goals—and yes, it may still be years away. The human kidney is incredibly complex, filtering nearly 50 gallons of blood a day, balancing electrolytes, managing hormones, and more—all in real time. Replacing that with a reliable, compact, and biocompatible device is no small feat.

But here's the good news: we've already come a long way. Just like it took only 66 years to go from the Wright brothers' first flight to Neil Armstrong's first step on the moon, the pace of progress is accelerating. Today we have advanced lab equipment, AI-powered diagnostics, bioengineering breakthroughs, and a growing global effort focused on kidney research.

The timeline may still be long, but we're no longer crawling. We're gaining altitude.

Appendix 3 - Fundraising Without Feeling Like A Burden

Worksheet for Planning with Purpose and Pride

A3.1 - What Feels Comfortable for You?

Fundraising comes in many forms. Check any options below that feel *right* for you:

☐ I'm okay asking directly
☐ I'd rather have someone else ask on my behalf
☐ I want to offer something in return (like a product or service)
☐ I prefer something low-key and personal
☐ I'd like to involve a group or community (church, work, school, etc.)

Your thoughts:

A3.2 - What's Your Story?

Use this space to write a few short lines you or someone else could use to explain your situation honestly and with dignity. It doesn't have to be perfect—just real.

- What you're facing:
- Why you're fundraising:
- How people can help:

(This can also be used as your intro for a social media post or donation page.)

Your thoughts:

A3.3 - What Could You Offer ?

Sometimes it helps to turn your fundraiser into an exchange. What could you give back to those who donate? Check or write your own notes:

☐ T-shirts or wristbands

☐ Baked goods or homemade items

☐ Art, poetry, or music

☐ Digital content (eBook, thank-you video, etc.)

☐ Event access (in-person or virtual)

☐ Personal note or update

☐ I'd rather just offer gratitude—nothing physical needed

List Your Ideas here:

A3.4 - Who Could Help You Share the Load?

Asking doesn't have to be a solo mission. List friends, family, coworkers, or community leaders who might help spread the word or organize a small event:

1

2

3

4

5

6

7

8

9

10

Final Thought

You're not asking for pity.
You're giving others the chance to **show up for you**.
That's not a burden—it's a gift.

Use the space below to write some notes and ideas to yourself.

Appendix 4 - Tips for Writing Request Letters

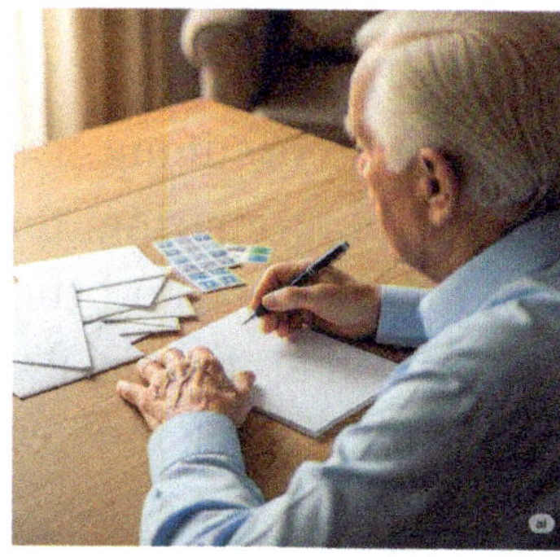

1. **Keep it simple and sincere:** Write as if you're speaking to someone who cares—and most do.
2. **Open with context:** Briefly share who you are and your connection to the group or leader.
3. **Name the challenge:** Be honest about your situation, but don't feel pressured to overshare medical details.
4. **Make the ask:** Be clear. What do you need, financial help, a fundraiser, a bulletin post, or prayer support?
5. **Express gratitude:** Thank them for their time and willingness to even consider your request.
6. **Offer follow-up:** Let them know you're happy to talk more, and include your contact info.
7. **Do follow ups:** Provide updates on your journey including any accomplishments.
8. **Thank you notes:** You might need to circle back later. A little gratitude now goes a long way When people feel appreciated, doors stay open. But when they feel used, those doors don't just close—they get dead-bolted with a chair jammed under the knob.

A4.1 - Sample Request Letter: Faith or Community Support

Subject: A Personal Request for Support

Dear [Pastor/Rabbi/Imam/Leader's Name],

I hope you're doing well. I wanted to share something personal—I'm preparing for a kidney transplant. I'm deeply grateful for the care and the path ahead. However, this journey comes with real financial strain: travel, temporary housing, recovery, and lifelong medications.

I'm doing my best to focus on healing, but I've come to realize that I can't do this alone. I'm reaching out to ask if there is any support available through our [church/temple/mosque/???], whether through a compassion fund, member outreach, or even just help spreading the word.

If it's fitting, I'd be honored to be included in a prayer list or have a moment shared in the announcements or bulletins. This isn't easy to ask—but I've come to see that asking for help is sometimes an act of faith, too.

Thank you for considering my request. Even a small bit of support—prayers, encouragement, or simply sharing my story—makes a big difference. I am happy to speak with you directly if you'd like.

With gratitude,

[Your Name]
[Phone or Email, if applicable]

A4.2 - Sample Request Letter: Union or Civic Club Support

Subject: Request for Member Assistance During Medical Recovery

Dear [Union President/Club Chair/Organization Leader],

My name is [Your Name], and I've been a [member/supporter/participant] of [Local #/Club Name] for [X] years. I'm reaching out during a challenging time to ask if there are any support programs or member resources available through the organization.

I'm currently preparing for a kidney transplant and facing some steep medical and travel-related costs. Between recovery time, income loss, and post-op care, it's been humbling to admit I could use a hand.

If there's a way the group could help—through a member fund, fundraiser, or even by sharing my story—I'd be incredibly grateful. I've always admired how this group looks after its own, and I'm leaning on that spirit of solidarity now.

Thank you for your time and consideration. I'd be happy to provide more details or speak directly if needed.

In solidarity,
[Your Name]
[Phone or Email]

A4.3 - Letter to a Nonprofit or Foundation (for support or publicity)

Subject: Request for Support or Awareness – Kidney Transplant Patient Outreach

Dear [Organization Name or Contact Person],

My name is [Your Name], and I'm reaching out as someone currently navigating the long road toward a kidney transplant. I've been managing end-stage kidney disease and am now advocating for myself while raising awareness about the realities patients face.

I'm writing to ask if your organization could help share my story, provide guidance, or connect me with any resources that might ease this journey. I'd also be grateful if you'd consider sharing my [link to GoFundMe/page/social media post] on your channels.

Thank you for the work you do. People like me truly benefit from it.

Sincerely,
[Your Full Name]
[Phone or Email]
[Link to transplant listing, GoFundMe, social page, etc.]

A4.4 Sample 2: Submission to a Local Newspaper or Community Blog

Subject: Local Resident Shares Real-Life Kidney Transplant Journey

Dear Editor,

My name is [Your Name], and I'm a local resident facing a medical challenge that affects thousands of Americans – end-stage kidney disease. I'm currently on the transplant list and navigating the ups, downs, and hopeful moments of this journey.

I'd love the opportunity to share a short article or letter with your readers about what it's like to walk this path, in hopes it might raise awareness, encourage living donation, or just connect with someone out there facing the same thing.

Please let me know if there's a space available for this kind of personal health story. I'd be honored to contribute.

Warm regards,
[Your Full Name]
[Contact info]

A4.5 - Pitch for a Blog or Health Advocacy Website

Subject: Personal Story Submission – Life on the Kidney Transplant List

Hi [Editor's Name or Website Team],

I've been following your blog and appreciate the real, human voices you feature. I'm currently on the kidney transplant list and wanted to submit a short personal story that reflects what this journey looks like from the patient side.

It's not all doom and gloom — there's humor, hope, and a fair amount of dialysis machine drama. I'd love to share something that speaks to others going through it and maybe even inspires a few people to consider living donation or organ registration.

I am happy to send over a 600–800 word draft for your review. Thanks for considering!

Best,
[Your First Name]
[Your Contact Info]
[Social or GoFundMe link if applicable]

A4.6 - Letter to a Healthcare Professional (for support or networking)

Subject: Patient Request – Guidance on Kidney Transplant Advocacy

Dear Dr. [Last Name] or [Transplant Coordinator's Name],

I hope this note finds you well. I'm one of your patients, currently being evaluated for a kidney transplant, and wanted to ask for some guidance on how best to advocate for myself during this time.

I'm looking into ways to share my story or spread awareness locally, and I'd appreciate any tips, contacts, or advice you might be able to share. I understand how busy things are and thank you in advance for any help you can offer.

Warmly,

[Your Name]
[Patient ID if needed]
[Phone or Email]

A4.8 - Letter to a Local Radio Host or Podcast

Subject: Possible Guest or Segment Idea – Real Kidney Transplant Journey

Hi [Host's Name],

I'm a local resident going through the process of finding a kidney donor and wanted to reach out in case this might be a topic of interest for your show.

This journey is filled with challenges and hope, and sharing it might help others understand the organ transplant process or even inspire a donor out there to step forward. I'd be honored to share my experience on air or even submit a short segment for you to consider.

Thanks so much for your time — and for keeping community voices alive on the airwaves.

Sincerely,
[Your Name]
[Contact Info]
[Optional: Website, page, or social media link]

A4.7 - Social Media DM or Post Message (Short + Shareable)

Hi friends,

As some of you know, I'm on the kidney transplant list and currently going through treatment. I'm sharing my story to help raise awareness — and maybe connect with someone who can help or just needs to hear they're not alone.

Please feel free to share this link: [insert GoFundMe, hospital listing, or transplant center page]

If you know of any blogs, news outlets, or community groups that might want to highlight a real-life transplant journey, I'd love an introduction. Thank you for reading and supporting.

Appendix 5 - Being A Living Donor

Note: This section isn't about guilt trips or pressure. It's about honesty. Living donation is a profound act with life-changing impact, and it deserves open, meaningful conversation. My goal here is to share a few facts and realities so people can understand what's truly involved.

While this book is primarily written for transplant recipients, it's worth pausing to shine a spotlight on the extraordinary people who make many transplants possible — living donors.

Living donors aren't superheroes in capes (though they deserve one). They're regular people — siblings, friends, co-workers, neighbors — who make an extraordinary choice to step up for someone else. Sometimes it's for a loved one they've known forever. Other times, it's for a complete stranger. Either way, the ripple effect of that decision is enormous: families get more time together, kids get more years with a parent, and entire communities feel the impact.

This section is about awareness. Because for every person who already knows they'd be willing to donate, there are many more who simply never knew it was possible, safe, and so desperately needed.

A5.1 - Why is it possible

Many people are surprised to learn that a healthy person can live a full, normal, and active life with just one kidney. Our bodies are built with some remarkable redundancy — like having a "spare" in case of emergency. In many cases, one well-functioning kidney can handle all the filtering and waste removal a body needs.

That's what makes living kidney donation not only possible, but life-changing. It's not science fiction. It's not a last-resort gamble. It's a safe, carefully planned medical process that can give someone years — even decades — of healthy life they might not otherwise have.

A5.2 - Number of patients on the lists

Based on data from various sources, the number of people on the kidney transplant waiting list in the United States is around **90,000 to 100,000**.

It's important to note this number changes daily as people are added and some receive transplants or are removed for various reasons, including changes in health status or even death.

The number of people waiting for a kidney transplant consistently represents over 85% of the total number of people on all the national organ transplant waiting lists.

A5.3 - Why Living Donation Matters

When someone needs a kidney transplant, they are placed on a national waiting list. Unfortunately, this list is incredibly long, with wait times that can span years—sometimes even a decade or more. For many patients, the wait is simply too long, and they may pass away before a suitable kidney becomes available. This is a heartbreaking reality across the U.S. and in many other countries.

This is where living kidney donation makes a profound difference. A kidney from a **living donor** can be transplanted much sooner, bypassing the lengthy wait on the deceased donor list. Beyond the significant reduction in wait time, these kidneys generally offer better long-term outcomes.

Kidneys from living donors often start working almost immediately and tend to function better and last longer than kidneys from **deceased donors**. This is because the organ is transplanted from a healthy living person, reducing the amount of time the kidney is outside the body (known as cold ischemia time) before transplantation. A shorter cold ischemia time is a key factor in improving the long-term success of the transplant.

A5.4 - What It Involves

Becoming a living donor isn't something to take lightly. **It's a serious commitment**, and the evaluation process is designed to be thorough for good reason: to protect the donor's health just as much as the recipient's.

Donors go have exams, lab work, imaging, and meet with social workers, psychologists, and transplant coordinators. The idea is to ensure that donating won't jeopardize the donor's physical or mental health and their well-being: short- or long-term.

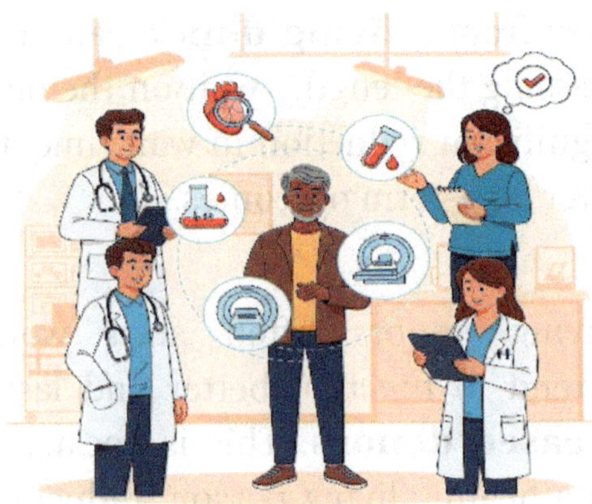

It's not just about compatibility. It's also about readiness, motivation, and support.

A5.5 - Costs and Challenges

Let's talk logistics. In most cases, the recipient's insurance, the transplant center or a charitable trust covers the medical costs related to the donation – testing, surgery, hospital stay, and follow-up.

But there are other costs donors may face, like lost wages during recovery, travel expenses, household expense or child care. These normally aren't covered. There are organizations and assistance programs that can help, but it takes planning and advocacy. See also fundraising: Appendix 3, for more insights and ideas.

Recovery time for a living donor is usually quicker than for a recipient, but it's still a big deal. Most healthy donors could return to work and regular life in about 6–8 weeks, though heavy lifting or strenuous activity may need to wait longer. That's because donation is still major surgery – the body needs time to heal inside and out. The donor should discuss their expected down time with the medical teams during evaluations.

While donors generally don't face the same months-long recovery or medication changes as recipients, they may still experience fatigue, soreness, or other healing challenges. Having solid support at home and understanding from employers makes a huge difference in how smoothly that recovery goes.

A5.6 - Exploring the Possibilities

If you (or someone you know) is curious about being a living donor – whether for a loved one or even a stranger – there are safe, thoughtful ways to explore it.

You can start by contacting your nearest transplant center and asking to speak to the living donor team. You can also check out organizations like the National Kidney Foundation or Living Donor Assistance Program to learn more.

A5.7 Saying No or Pausing

Donors can say no at any time, and they should never feel pressured. Even after passing all the requirements and joining the donor list, you have the right to remove yourself.

Life changes—whether it's a shift in circumstances, work, or health—can make donation not the right choice at that moment or not at all. Saying no isn't backing down; it's a responsible and courageous decision.

A5.8 Let's Break the Silence

Most folks don't even know living kidney donation is a thing—I know I had never heard about it until I ended up needing a transplant myself.

It's one of those topics that doesn't get talked about enough, or even at all. Just by sharing what you've learned, by opening up the conversation with your family, friends, or community, you could be planting a seed. That seed might grow into someone stepping up to say "yes" when it really matters.

Talking openly about living kidney donation is powerful. By simply sharing the facts and stories, you help remove the stigma and fear that keep people from learning more. When we speak up, we create space for understanding and hope — and maybe inspire someone else to take that life-saving step when they're ready.

In Closing

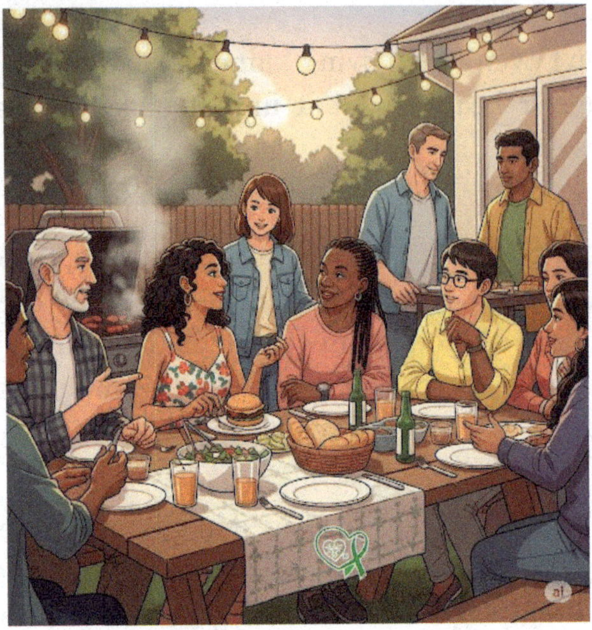

Remember, you don't have to be ready or even eligible to donate yourself, by learning about living donation and sharing that knowledge helps spread awareness. Your voice might inspire someone else to say "yes" when the time is right.

So don't underestimate the power of simply talking about it. You never know whose life you might touch.

Appendix 6 – Transferring to a New Transplant Center

Your ability to move and transfer to another transplant center for on going care can be summed up into one word: **<u>MAYBE</u>**.

If this is something you are considering or want to explore, here are a few of the steps you must think about. This only some general ones to be aware of before you book a moving truck.

Some important steps:

- Notify Your Current Transplant Center and Doctors
- Research New Transplant Centers and Specialists
- Coordinate that everyone is ready to go to receive you
- Transfer Medical Records and Test Results
- Coordinate Your Medication Supply
- Schedule Your First Appointments in the New Location
- Update Your Health Insurance and Contact Information
- Plan for Emergency Care
- Arrange Support Services
- Monitor Your Health Closely During Transition

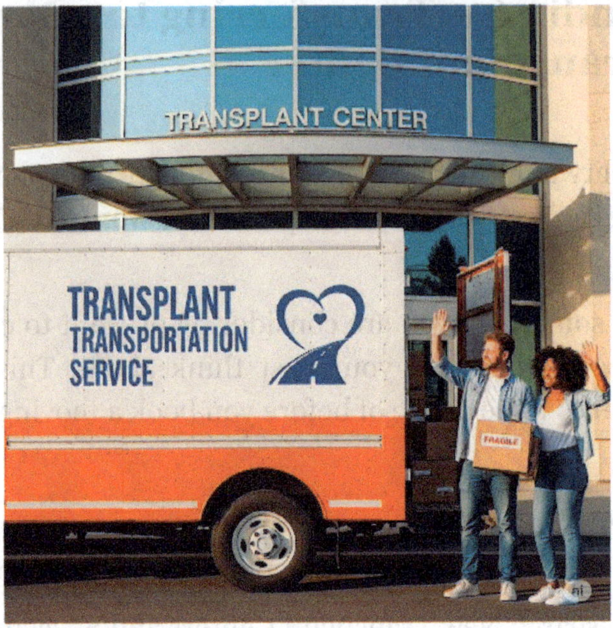

A6.1 - The Conversation Starts Early

The first and most important step is simple: talk to your current transplant team first. They'll need to help coordinate the move with your new center. They might even have a list of trusted transplant centers in the area you're heading to.

Your current team will be the ones handling the heavy lifting—like preparing and transferring your medical records—so looping them in early makes everything smoother. You can not do this solo. They are your best ally in making the transition safe and seamless. And even possible.

A6.2 - The Insurance Puzzle

This is a critical, and often complex, piece of the puzzle. You need to verify that your current and new insurance will cover your care at the new transplant center and with the new doctors. This is a potential deal-breaker.

You should:

- **Contact your insurance provider** to understand what their policies are for out-of-state transplant care. You may have to completely sign up with another company if your carrier does not operate in the new state or their plans in the new state are not compatible with your requirements.
- **Check with the new transplant center's financial coordinator** to ensure your insurance is accepted and what your out-of-pocket costs might be.
- **If on Medicare/Medicaid** – you will need verify if you are even eligible to change states.

A6.4 - The Kidney Specialist (Nephrologist)

A new kidney specialist must agree to take you on. This is often the trickiest part, as many specialists have long patient lists. You need to find a new nephrologist who is not only a good fit for you but also affiliated with your receiving transplant center. The new transplant center's team may have a list of nephrologists they recommend or work with closely.

A6.3 - The New Transplant Center's Vetting Process

Because of the burden they are assuming, not all transplant centers may be as willing to accept external patients. Their staff may already be short handed and unable to support additional patients and the associated obligations.

Think of this as the application process all over again. The new transplant center won't just accept your current doctor's recommendation; they will conduct their own thorough review.

This typically involves:

- **A full review of your medical history:** The new team will want every detail of your transplant and recovery.

- **Your own evaluation:** They may require you to undergo some of the same tests you had before your transplant, such as blood work or imaging, to establish a baseline in their system.

- **A meeting with their team:** You will likely meet with the social workers, financial coordinators, nephrologist team, and transplant coordinator to ensure everyone is on the same page. You understand their program's specific rules and expectations.

A6.6 - The "Trees in the Wind" Rules

Each transplant center has its own unique set of rules. This can include:

- **Medication protocols:** While the core drugs might be the same, the dosages or specific brands might vary.
- **Follow-up schedule:** The frequency and type of check-ins could be different.
- **Support systems:** They may have different expectations for your support network.

And time. Budget lots of time. Months are entirely possible.

And money. Maybe lots of money. You may have to travel in advance to the new clinic and meet with team members before they will even consider your application. And you might have to return for testings/screenings. Tests and specialists who are NOT covered by your current insurance.

In short

A move to a new transplant center is a very real possibility, but it's not a simple transfer. It's more of a restart of the evaluation process with a new team. The key is to be proactive, communicate constantly with both teams, and be prepared for a thorough re-evaluation.

Appendix 7 - Safety in Seconds — Medical ID and Document Access

A7.1 - Tags, Docs, and Lockboxes — Staying Ready, Staying Safe

As you've seen throughout this handbook, transplant success is more than surgery and medication—it's staying informed, prepared, and empowered. The journey doesn't end at discharge. It continues with you every day: how you communicate your needs, how you protect your health, and how you ensure your wishes are respected in any situation.

In this appendix, I will cover two often-overlooked tools in that journey: **medical identification** and **secure access to legal and medical documents**. Whether you're simply navigating a new hospital system, traveling, or unconscious, having the right information visible and accessible can make all the difference.

From bracelets that speak for you when you can't, to digital lockboxes that outsmart the filing cabinet, this section is your cheat sheet for staying safe and sane when the unexpected hits.

- Medical IDs alert responders to your transplant status, allergies, and care needs.
- Legal documents guide treatment when you can't speak for yourself.
- Secure access prevents delays, errors, and unwanted interventions.

A7.1 - Medical ID Options

Choose what fits your lifestyle and comfort level. All should include transplant status and emergency contact info.

Type	*Description*	*Notes*
Bracelet	*Durable, engraved, visible*	*Stainless steel or silicone*
Dog Tags	*Necklace-style, discreet*	*Can include multiple tags*
Wallet Card	*Paper or plastic, detailed*	*Include physician contact*
QR Code Tag	*Links to secure online profile*	*HIPAA-compliant platforms available*

I have bracelets and 'dog tags'.

Line 1: Left Arm No B/P or I/V

Line 2: Kidney Transplant

Line 3: U of Mich Patient ID No.

Line 4: Name / Blood Type / Organ Donor

Because surface can eventually wear down, the engraving may be unreadable even with a bright light. I get new ones every couple of years.

A7.3 Legal & Medical Documents

These guide your care when you can't speak for yourself. Keep them updated and accessible.

- Advance Directive / Living Will
- Durable Power of Attorney for Health Care
- POLST (Physician Orders for Life-Sustaining Treatment)
- DNR (Do Not Resuscitate)
- Transplant-specific instructions (e.g., medication alerts, dialysis history)

A7.3.1 - The Problem with Too Many Copies

- Hospitals often want their own version
- Family members may misplace or forget updates
- Updating means tracking down every copy
- More copies = more risk of outdated or conflicting info

A7.3.2 - Smart Solutions for Secure Access

A7.3.2.1 Nevada's Lockbox System

A free, state-run registry for advance directives and guardianship nominations.

- Hosted by the Nevada Secretary of State
- Secure online access for hospitals and courts
- Patients receive a wallet card with registration number
- Easy to update — no need to resend copies

https://www.nvsos.gov/sos/online-services/nevada-lockbox

A7.3.2.2 - Other Options by State or Platform

Option	*Description*	*Pros*	*Cons*
State Registries	*Arizona, Oregon, and others offer directive registries*	*Centralized, official*	*Not universal*
Online Vaults	*MyDirectives, Everplans, Cake*	*Easy to share, update*	*May charge fees*
USB Medical Tags	*Flash drive with encrypted docs*	*Portable*	*Risk of loss*
Cloud + QR Code	*Google Drive, Dropbox + QR tag*	*Flexible*	*Requires tech setup*

A7.3.3 Best Practices

- Choose one secure method and stick with it
- Limit copies to 2–3 trusted people or providers
- Review annually or after major health changes
- Use a medical ID that references your document access method *(e.g., "See QR tag for directive")*

Closing Summary: Stay Ready, Stay Protected

Your transplant journey is built on resilience, trust, and preparation. While medical ID and document access may seem like small details, they can make a life-saving difference when time is short and decisions are critical. Whether you choose a bracelet, a QR tag, or a secure digital vault, the goal is simple: make sure the right people have the right information at the right time.

You don't need to do everything at once. Just start with one step —and build from there.

Quick Checklist: Your Emergency Readiness Toolkit

[ ] Choose a medical ID (bracelet, dog tag, wallet card, or QR tag)

[ ] Include transplant status and emergency contact info

[ ] Gather key documents (Advance Directive, POA, POLST, DNR)

[ ] Select a secure access method (state registry, online vault, cloud link)

[ ] Limit copies to 2–3 trusted people or providers

[ ] Review and update annually

[ ] Inform your care team where to find your documents

[ ] Keep a backup (digital or physical) in a known location

May the insights within these pages prepare you not just for a transplant, but for renewal, resilience, and the life waiting beyond.

—John Carter

Made in the USA
Monee, IL
12 September 2026

62981018R00154